ULCERATIVE COLITIS – TREATMENTS, SPECIAL POPULATIONS AND THE FUTURE

Edited by **Mortimer O'Connor**

Ulcerative Colitis – Treatments, Special Populations and the Future
Edited by Mortimer O'Connor

Published by InTech
Janeza Trdine 9, 51000 Rijeka, Croatia

Publishing Process Manager Danijela Duric

Technical Editor Teodora Smiljanic

Cover Designer InTech Design Team

Additional hard copies can be obtained from orders@intechopen.com

Ulcerative Colitis – Treatments, Special Populations and the Future,
Edited by Mortimer O'Connor
p. cm.
ISBN 978-953-307-739-0

For EU product safety concerns:
IN TECH d.o.o., Prolaz Marije Krucifikse Kozulić 3, 51000 Rijeka, Croatia,
info@intechopen.com or visit our website at intechopen.com.

Meet the editor

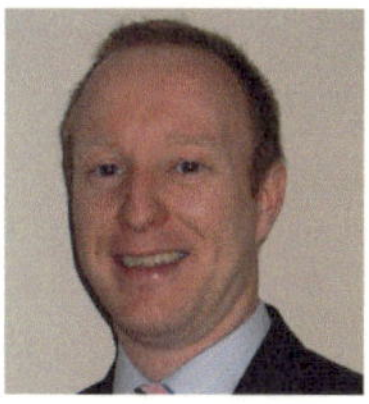

Dr O'Connor, who is a native of Cork in Ireland, achieved entry to read Medicine at University College Cork in 2001 with an academic scholarship. He graduated in 2006 and has since pursued a career in the field of Clinical Medicine with an ever growing interest in Clinical Research. He has worked clinically in the areas of Gastroenterology, Infectious Disease, Rheumatology, Oncology, along with many other specialties. He currently holds the position of Medical Registrar at the South Infirmary Victoria University Hospital, Cork, Ireland, where he is co-founder and co-chair of the "Dr John Walsh Research Foundation". He is an author on more than 100 published medical papers and is an active reviewer for several national and international journals. His publications cover many areas from Gastroenterology, Infectious Disease, Rheumatology, Neurology and Vaccines to Medical Communication skills. This is his first position as Book Editor.

Contents

Preface

Gastroenterology is the branch of medicine whereby the digestive system and its disorders are studied. The name is a combination of three Ancient Greek words *gaster* (*gastros or stomach), enteron* (intestine), and *logos* (reason). Its documented history dates back to Egyptian times where, citing from Egyptian papyri, Nunn identified significant knowledge of gastrointestinal diseases among practicing physicians during the periods of the pharaohs, while Irynakhty, of the tenth dynasty, c. 2125 B.C., was a court physician specializing in gastroenterology and proctology. Among ancient Greeks, Hippocrates attributed digestion to concoction, while Galen's concept of the stomach having four *faculties* was widely accepted up to modernity in the seventeenth century. Since then the works of Maximilian Stroll in 1777 (described cancer of the gallbladder), Karl Wilhelm von Kupffer in 1876 (described the properties of liver Kupffer cells), Burrill Bernard Crohn in 1932 (described Crohn's disease), and Barry Marshall, Robin Warren and James Leavitt in 1982/1983 (discovery of Helicobacter pylori and its role in peptic ulcer disease), to mention just a few, has evolved the thinking of gastroenterology. It is clearly seen by the history of Gastroenterology the speciality continues to develop at a rapid pace due to growth in the understanding of disease processes and the discovery of new diagnostic and treatment strategies. Ulcerative Colitis is no exception to this trend. This book is just another step in marking the current developing knowledge and thinking around the area of Ulcerative colitis.

This book, which comes in two volumes, is intended to act as an up to date reference point and knowledge developer for all readers interested in the area of gastroenterology and in particular Ulcerative Colitis. All of the chapter authors are experts in their fields of publication and deserve individual credit and praise for their contributions to this book. We hope that you will find this publication informative, stimulating and a reference point for the area of Ulcerative colitis as we move forward in our understanding of the field of medicine. With that hope, I remind you of the though provoking quote by the French Philosopher and writer, Voltaire (1694 – 1778), *"Doctors are men who prescribe medicines of which they know little, to cure disease of which they know less, in human beings of whom they know nothing".*

Acknowledgements

Many thanks to the authors of each Chapter of this book. The outstanding contributions they have made resulted in a very easy book to edit. It was very enjoyable and a privilege reading each contribution. Your work is now a mark for the future.

To the publisher, InTech, thank you for being ever present and encouraging me in my endeavors to stay up to date with the review and editing process. I would never have been so organized without the assistance of Ms. Danijela Duric, Publishing Process Manager. It was a pleasure to edit my first book with such a wonderful group.

To my father (Tim) and late mother (Eileen), thank you for all the encouragement over the years to achieve my goals and become the ever developing doctor that I am today. I could not have achieved a fraction of my success without the support and love. Mam, I know you are always watching over and guiding me from a place nearby.

Dr Catherine O'Connor, my late aunt, who was always an inspiration. The ever present support and guidance in my early years of life and career where far beyond the role of an aunt or godmother. You will always be an example of professionalism I will strive to achieve.

Finally, to my other half, Bernie. All those long evenings spent without me while I was reading chapters and doing background knowledge discovery for this book are finally over. Your support is always beyond the call of duty and appreciated. Thank you.

Mortimer B. O'Connor
Department of Medicine, South Infirmary Victoria University Hospital,
Old Blackrock Road, Cork
Ireland

Part 1

Treatments

1

Surgical Treatment of Ulcerative Colitis

Gianluca Pellino[1], Guido Sciaudone[1], Gabriele Riegler[2],
Silvestro Canonico[1] and Francesco Selvaggi[1]
[1]General Surgery Unit
[2]Division of Gastroenterology
Second University of Naples
Italy

1. Introduction

Ulcerative colitis (UC) is an ubiquitously distributed inflammatory bowel disease. Its incidence varies slightly between geographical areas, most likely because of either the different genetic patrimonies of the involved populations or several environmental factors. In socially evolved Countries UC incidence is of approximately 6 cases per 100.000 white adult individuals, with a prevalence of 40-100/100.000. This incidence notably decreases in Countries with lower socio-economic levels. Female gender is slightly more affected than male, with a gender ratio F/M of 1.5/1.

The aetiology of UC still remains mainly unknown, even if a multifactorial genesis is now widely accepted.

Unlike Crohn's disease, UC is a continuous disease involving mainly the rectum, suddenly expanding proximally to the colon, with no alternation of healthy or diseased mucosal area. Figure 1 depicts the possible localization of UC at the time of clinical presentation (Binder et al., 1982; Stonnington et al., 1987)

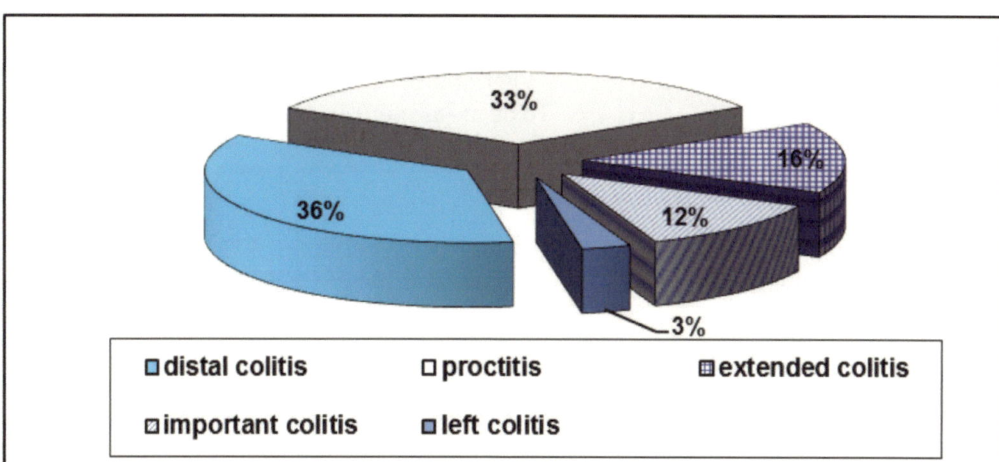

Fig. 1. Extension of ulcerative colitis at presentation

In case of pancolitis, in about 10-20% of patients also the last 5-15 cm of distal ileum can be involved, with ulcerated lesions of the mucosa, pathologically undistinguishable from colon lesions, picture defined as *backwash ileitis.* Disease usually presents with an acute attack or with a relapse in patients with an history of muco-haematic diarrhoea (Edwards & Truelove, 1963).
Even if only the complete removal of involved organs - colon and rectum - ensures complete recovery, the treatment of UC is, initially, mainly medical, based on drugs such as corticosteroids, salicylates, immunomodulators, and, more recently, biologics.
However, between 20 and 40% of patients will require surgery (Leijonmarck et al., 1990). Extension of the disease represents an important factor influencing treatment choice. In fact, only 2% of patients with a disease confined to the rectum require surgery during the 5 years after the diagnosis, whereas 35% of patients with pancolitis will be operated on (Richie, 1974).
Indications to surgery consist of complications, such as toxic megacolon, perforation, hemorrhage, presence of intractable extra-intestinal manifestations, risk of carcinoma, and failure of medical treatment.
During years, surgical treatment of UC has dramatically changed, even if still ensuring disease eradication. In fact, giving an alternative to proctococolectomy with definitive ileostomy, option very humiliating for the patient, Parks and Nicholls (Parks & Nicholls, 1978) proposed in 1978 the *restorative proctocolectomy* (RP), fashioning an ileal reservoir (*pouch*) that offered patients a radical treatment of the disease but also a good anal function, preserving intestinal continuity and the anus in its natural site. This intervention, consisting of removal of the entire colon and rectum to the *linea dentata,* hence preserving the sphincters, followed by fashioning of a neo-rectum with the last ileal loops and ileo-anal anastomosis, represented a revolution in surgical treatment of UC, rapidly becoming the intervention of choice for UC in selected centres (Pemberton et al., 1987; Williams, 1989; Selvaggi et al., 1996)

2. Indications to surgery

Indications to surgical treatment of UC can be distinguished in indications to elective and emergency - relative or absolute - surgery (Table 1).

Elective surgery	Absolute emergency	Relative emergency
Failure of medical therapy Extraintestinal manifestations Preventing degeneration	Perforation Toxic megacolon	Hemorrhage Severe colitis

Table 1. Indications to surgical treatment of UC

The rate of patients at risk of experiencing an acute complication of UC (perforation, toxic megacolon, hemorrhage, severe colitis) ranges between 10 and 20% (Jewell, 1987; Truelove, 1988).

2.1 Perforation

It usually occurs in patients presenting with dilatation of the colon. It represents an absolute indication to surgical intervention in emergency settings and tends to occur soon during the course of the disease, before bowel thickening. Incidence of perforation is reported to be as high as 3% (Kirsner & Shorter, 1982)

2.2 Toxic megacolon

It occurs in 5-10% of patients (with perforation 0.9-1.6%) (Kirsner & Shorter, 1982). Bowel dilatation >6 cm represents an absolute indication to surgery. In such patients a subtotal colectomy with closure of the rectal stump and Brooke terminal ileostomy is recommended.

2.3 Hemorrhage

It is a rare complication (3%), that can usually be managed with medical treatment or with rectal washout with adrenaline in saline solution (1/200.000). If it is not possible, there is indication to surgery; it should be considered, however, that haemorrhage can continue in the residual rectum, if a subtotal colectomy is performed (12%) (Kirsner & Shorter, 1982).

2.4 Severe colitis

An acute episode of colitis is defined *severe* if bowel movements with blood are more than 6 in 24 hours, median afternoon temperature is >37.5°C or median entire day temperature is >37.7°C at least 2 out of 4 days, hearth rate is >90 bpm, ESR is >30, Hb is <10 g/dL. Such a condition, occurring in 10-15% of patients (Truelove & Jewell, 1974), requires intensive medical therapy with correction of hydro-electrolytic disturbances, albumin and corticosteroid infusion, plasma and/or blood infusion, total parenteral nutrition. Treatment should be tried for a maximum of 5 days; if there is no improvement of patient condition, emergency colectomy is required (Truelove & Witts, 1955; Turnbull et al., 1971). Most Authors believe, however, that if a plain abdominal radiograph documents colonic dilatation >6/7 cm or mucosal islands, surgical intervention should be performed after 24 hours of ineffective therapy at most (Bartram, 1987). In 1975 Lennard-Jones (Lennard-Jones et al., 1975) suggested some parameters predicting poor response to medical treatment (Table 2).

Factor	% Failure
Bowel movements > 9/24h	33
Bowel movements > 12/24h	55
Temperature > 38 °C	56
Albumin < 3 g/dl	42
Mucosal islands on plain adbominal rx	75

Table 2. Factors predicting poor response to medical treatment

2.5 Failure of medical therapy

It probably represents the most common indication to surgery.

In patients with debilitating symptoms, a poor nutritional condition and an unsatisfactory quality of life despite adequate medical therapy, the eventuality of an elective surgical intervention should be considered. Some Authors (Mitchell et al., 1988) suggested that a prolonged medical treatment could increase the probability of surgery in emergency settings with consequential increase of morbidity, hospital stay and costs. Moreover, the prolonged medical treatment which UC patients often need, can have important secondary effects such as psychosis, hypertension, cataract, osteoporosis, insomuch as some Authors (Sagar et al., 1993) report a better quality of life in patients undergoing RP than in those receiving prolonged medical treatment.

2.6 Extraintestinal manifestations

About 30% of UC patients have at least one extraintestinal manifestation contributing to opt for surgery. Some manifestations, such as those involving skin, distal joints, eyes, or hematologic and vascular ones, can improve after surgery, whereas some other like pyoderma gangrenosum, ankylosing spondilytis, and rheumatoid arthritis do not seem to be modified by surgical intervention.

2.7 Prevention of neoplastic degeneration

Factors predisposing to colorectal cancer in UC patients consist of pancolitis, duration of disease, active disease and its severity. Early UC onset is another independent risk factor.
Beside these factors, dysplasia represents the precancerous lesion from which colorectal cancer subsequently arise (Morson, 1962; Morson & Pang, 1967).
In fact, > 70% of patients with colorectal cancer on UC have dysplasia on colorectal mucosa (Taylor et al., 1992; Connell et al., 1994). Severe dysplasia is reported to develop colorectal cancer in 45% of cases, whereas there are too few data in literature to do a similar valuation for mild-moderate dysplasia (Collins et al., 1987; Bernestein et al.,1994).
Furthermore, the risk of colorectal cancer is due to the evidence that high grade dysplasia represents a marker of cancer in another colon site in 45% of patients (Provenzale et al.,1995).
A review analyzing 116 studies pointed out that the global risk for colorectal cancer in UC patients is 8% after 20 years of disease, increasing gradually during years (Table 3), with a global rate of 3.7% (Van Heerden et al., 1980).

Risk (%)	Duration of disease (ys)
2	10
8	20
18	30

Table 3. Risk of colorectal cancer and duration of disease

This risk is approximately 8 times higher than normal population, increasing to 20 times if pancolitis is present; it is 4 times higher in case of left colitis (Gyde et al., 1988).
For these reasons, some Authors advocated prophylactic colectomy in UC patients affected from more than 10 years, but this approach is still matter of debate (Provenzale et al.,1995).

3. Surgical options

The possible surgical strategies can be schematized in three types of intervention:

- total proctocolectomy with definitive ileostomy
- total colectomy with ileo-rectal anastomosis (IRA)
- restorative proctocolectomy with ileal pouch (RP)

In 1997 Little and Parks (Little & Parks, 1977) proposed proctocolectomy with definitive ileostomy for the treatment of UC. This intervention surely gives the advantage of being curative, ensuring complete disease removal with a single intervention. Moreover such intervention, if intersphincteric proctectomy is performed and perianal skin closed, allows to reduce morbidity of rectal excision with its major complications, such as urinary and sexual dysfunctions and leakage due to the presence of anal canal. Definitive ileostomy with lost anorectal function is the principal drawback of this procedure. Ileostomy, in fact, determines an important handicap for the patient who feels permanently ill, and can cause

alteration of body image leading to depression, isolation and impairment of social function in 45% of patients (Skarsgard et al., 1989; Druss et al., 1968).
Total colectomy with ileo-rectal anastomosis proposed by Devine (Devine, 1943) and Corbett (Corbett, 1952) seems to avoid this problem because it does not require ileostomy, restoring intestinal continuity with ileo-rectal anastomosis. Furthermore, this intervention is able to ensure good results with low incidence of mortality - especially if performed in elective settings - and low incidence of anastomotic leakage and pelvic sepsis (Jones et al., 1977). The main advantage is that the preservation of anorectal function is possible avoiding genito-urinary dysfunctions due to proctectomy, with 4/5 evacuation/day. However, in a study from the Mayo Clinic involving 63 patients with IRA only 55% of patients was satisfied with function in the long term (Farnell & Adson, 1985). Moreover, about 1/3 of patients still need enemas with corticosteroids or sulfasalazine (Khubchandani et al., 1978).
Colectomy with IRA does not remove the entire diseased organ, and the preservation of the rectum rises the risk of late carcinogenesis or of severe proctitis, which can affect long term results of the intervention and require subsequent proctectomy in 5-30% of patients (Parc et al., 1989). The presence of carcinoma, severe rectal disease and incompetence of the sphincters represent absolute contraindications to colectomy with IRA.
For these reasons, researchers felt the need of perform interventions that could not only be curative and radical, but able to preserve sphincters and, therefore, an acceptable anal function.
To fulfill these aims, Parks and Nicholls (Parks & Nicholls, 1978) first described RP with ileal pouch in 1978, consisting of total colectomy, proximal proctectomy, mucosectomy of the distal rectum and ileopouch-anal anastomosis. The intervention which they proposed implied fashioning of an S-shaped ileal reservoir with three folded ileal loops anastomized to the anal canal after mucosectomy of the rectal stump toward the *linea pettinata*.
Subsequently Utsonomiya (Utsonomiya et al., 1980) perfectioned this reservoir, as it had important emptying problems due to the often excessive length of the efferent limb (about 5 cm), responsible for failure of spontaneous evacuation. In 1980 the Author proposed a J-shaped reservoir fashioned with two loops of small bowel. J-pouch, easy to perform even with mechanical staplers, avoided problems of S-pouch but it still comported an high number of evacuations, particularly during the first years after ileostomy reversal, hence in 1984 Nicholls (Nicholls & Pezim, 1984) suggested a new type of reservoir, fashioned with four ileal loops, the W-pouch, which assumed an almost spherical shape and seemed to offer a better evacuating function than J-pouch even if technically more difficult to fashion (Figure 2).
A study from the St. Mark's Hospital (Nicholls & Pezim, 1985) comparing W-, S- and J-pouch for frequency of evacuations reported an inverse correlation between frequency and maximum volume of the pouch: reservoir capacity is thus one of the main factors affecting defecation frequency and volume seems to be more relevant than shape. A sufficiently capable J-pouch - fashioned with two loops of approximately 20 cm each - could hence have results similar to those of W- or S-pouch.
In a prospective randomized trial Selvaggi et al.(Selvaggi et al., 2000) found that patients with J-pouch had an higher number of defecations than W-pouch in the short term; it should be noted, however, that after this initial difference J-pouch allows a number of evacuations similar to that of W-pouch in the long term.
In the description of their original technique Parks and Nicholls (Parks & Nicholls, 1978) described mucosectomy of the rectal stump toward the *linea pettinata* and ileopouch-anal

anastomosis at that level. This was regarded as a fundamental time of the procedure, allowing complete removal of the diseased tissue and definitive disease healing.

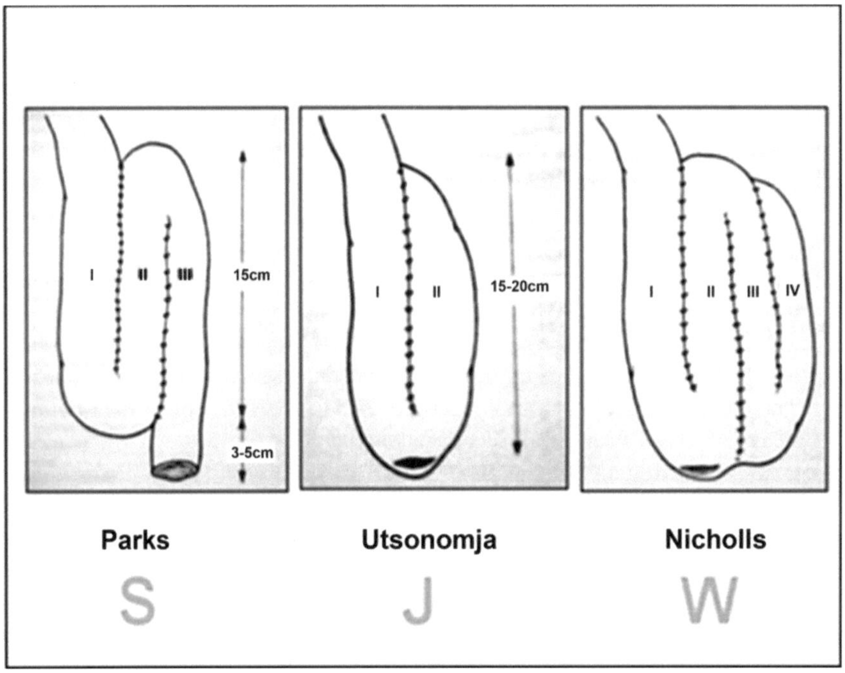

Fig. 2. Pouch configurations

Nowadays most Authors agree that preserving the rectum is useless, so it is sectioned at the level of anorectal junction. The preparation of the rectum toward anorectal junction is usually intramesorectal, which rises the risk of bleeding but also reduces the risk of nerve lesions. However mesorectal excision is mandatory in case of either severe dysplasia or cancer.

After pouch construction, ileopouch-anal anastomosis can be either manual or stapled. When mucosectomy is performed, it is necessary to fashion manual ileoanal anastomosis intra-anally by suturing the pouch to the anus with some stiches between it and the *linea dentata*. Mechanical anastomosis is performed with a circular stapled inserted trans-anally.

Mucosectomy guarantees complete eradication of the disease, avoiding both bleeding from persistent inflammation (Keighley et al.,1991), found in about 23% of cases (44%), and incidence of mucosal dysplasia and cancer development, but it is not routinely performed for several reasons: it is quite difficult to perform; it requires longer operatory times; it brings about risks of sphincter lesions both direct and due to anal divaricator; it can be difficult to get the apex of the pouch to the perineal plane to effectuate the anastomosis without tension; there is the risk of pelvic septic complications. Moreover, mucosectomy also removes anal transitional zone (AZT) which has sensitive function and contributes to perfect continence.

To avoid such problems a technique was proposed, consisting of section of the rectum about 2 cm above the *linea dentata* and stapled pouch-anal anastomosis. Further resection of 1 cm of rectum effectuated by the stapler poses the anastomosis just above the superior margin of the anal canal, with no need of mucosectomy.

As now, J- and W-pouch are the most used reservoirs, while S-pouch is not commonly performed due to the need of catheterization to facilitate evacuation in about 50% of patients.

Thus, RP represented a revolution in surgical treatment of UC, becoming in few years the intervention of choice in selected centers, as it allows a complete disease removal preserving intestinal continuity and the anus in its natural site, therefore ensuring good fecal continence and acceptable number of evacuation during one day. Moreover the simplification of the original procedure due to mechanical staplers to perform ileo-anal anastomosis significantly contributed to the diffusion of the technique.

The number of interventions necessary to perform RP can vary. In case of emergency settings, when patients usually are in severe general conditions, it is preferable to perform a total colectomy, postposing proctectomy and pouch construction. On the other hand, immunomodulators and, more recently, biologics demonstrated their effectiveness in controlling acute UC attack, allowing RP in elective settings when there is no absolute indication to surgery.

4. Patients selection

RP is nowadays the intervention of choice for surgical treatment of UC in so much that Dozois, already in 1988, stated that results with RP were so good that it should be preferred in the majority of patients.

Reliability of this intervention induced to extend surgical indication not only for patient with intractable UC but also for those in acceptable general conditions.

However, some factors should be considered before proposing to patients a RP.

First, diagnosis of UC must be histologically confirmed; if there is suspicion of Crohn's disease RP should be avoided, as Crohn's brings about a risk of perineal complications of about 50% with a 20-40% rate of pouch defunctioning/removal (Parker & Nicholls, 1991; Hyman et al., 1991).

Moreover a manometric examination of the sphincters must be carried out, because patients with poor sphincter function do not fit ileopouch-anal anastomosis.

Elderly represents a relative contraindication to RP: this is not due to patients' general health status, but to the more frequent incidence of fecal incontinence in the older population. In fact, anal contraction diminishes in over 70-year-old patients.

Patients already undergone anal surgery before RP have similar functional results than who did not (Selvaggi et al., 2010a).

RP is more difficult in patient with a small pelvis and in thin patients, as it could be difficult to get the pouch reach the anus without tension, even when all the techniques of mesenteric lengthening are performed. Obesity has represented another relative contraindication to RP, but the intervention is nowadays performed routinely also in obese patients.

Cancer of the colon or of the proximal rectum does not represent a contraindication to RP as it can be completely excised. When a locally invasive cancer with metastasis to regional nodes is diagnosed, total colectomy should be performed and adjuvant therapy should be given before proctectomy and pouch construction; in patients with metastatic disease RP is contraindicated and colectomy with IRA should be preferred.

5. Complications

Intraoperative mortality is reported to be lower than 1%, while global morbidity ranges between 13 and 54% after RP (Hosie et al., 1992; Metcalf et al., 1988; Nicholls & Pezim, 1984; Nicholls, 1993). Complications can occur early, after ileostomy closure or late.

5.1 Small bowel occlusion

It is an early complication occurring in 15% of patients before ileostomy closure. About 1/3 of these patients require surgical intervention. However, this rate is similar to that of other surgical interventions for UC. The rate of small bowel occlusion can reach 20-25% after ileostomy closure, so it is significantly higher than that after colectomy with terminal ileostomy (Marcello, 1993).

5.2 Pelvic sepsis

Manifestations of pelvic sepsis include abscess, flegmon and fistula. In the past this complication was reported to occur in 20-30% of patients, while nowadays its incidence dramatically reduced to 5-7% (Selvaggi et al., 2010b; Williams & Johnstone, 1985). Such a difference is probably due to both growing surgical experience and to complete rectal removal avoiding mucosectomy of a long rectal stump (Lohmuller et al., 1990). Some Authors reported that pelvic sepsis is a treating condition because, after its resolution, when the pouch is not excised, it determines pelvic fibrosis potentially affecting pouch compliance and, consequently, impair function.

5.3 Stenosis of ileopouch-anal anastomosis

Its incidence varies between 4 and 38%, being more frequent in case of stapled anastomosis. It is one of the most common causes of pouch malfunctioning due to the possibility of an outlet obstruction that can require several dilatations with Hegar dilators or, less frequently, redo-pouch (Nicholls, 1993).

5.4 Genito-urinary dysfunctions

They occur in approximately 11% of male and 12%of female (Nicholls, 1993). They are usually due to nerve lesions during rectal dissection and ligation of inferior mesenteric vessels and to post-surgical adhesions, that, in female gender, can cause infertility.
However, pregnancy is possible after RP.

5.5 Pouchitis

It is a common complication of RP. Diagnosis consists of contemporaneous presence of abdominal pain, emission of liquid feces with blood, urgency, incontinence, general malaise, and fever. Pathological confirmation is required with histological evidence of the inflammation. When all these criteria are satisfied, it has an incidence of 10%.
The risk of developing pouchitis is higher during the first 6 months after intervention; cumulative risk at 4 years is 51%, but <10% of patients present with a severe pouchitis and only 1.3% will require pouch excision; in most cases (90%) pouchitis presents with sporadic episodes, easily managed with metronidazole and, sometimes, enemas with steroids or 5-ASA. In the rare eventuality of intractable pouchitis a temporary ileostomy or pouch removal can be necessary (Lohmuller et al., 1990; Patel et al.,1995).

An increase in bowel frequency or a *malfunctioning* pouch are not enough to define pouchitis, but this is a common mistake.
We have recently demonstrated that COX-2 and VEGF are overexpressed in ileal pouch mucosa, potentially playing a role in development of pouchitis (Romano et al., 2007).

5.6 Malfunctioning pouch

Reasons determining a poor pouch function are various and, often, due to surgeon's experience.
They are often due to fashioning of pouch either too small, unable to fulfill reservoir function, or too big, unable to empty completely.
Causes determining pouch dysfunction can be classified on the basis of anatomic site which they originate from (Table 4) (Selvaggi et al., 2002).

Proximal ileum	Pouch	Outlet
Chronic obstruction Gut infections Alimentation Small bowel motility	Crohn's disease Indetermined colitis Shape Volume Peri-pouch fibrosis	Stenosis of pouch-anal anastomosis Pouch angulation Pouch torsion Long rectal stump Pouch prolapse Anal sphincters spasms Paradox contraction of puborectalis m.

Table 4. Causes of dysfunction and anatomic site

6. Conclusions

Aim of surgical treatment of UC is the complete removal of the disease. Indications to surgery in election are not, as now, better defined than they were in the past, because of both better knowledge of clinical history and more accurate prevention of an eventual neoplastic transformation obtained with pancolonoscopy with multiple bioptic sampling. On the other hand, nowadays more patients are operated on because recent procedures allow sphincters preservation and particularly to interposition of an ileal pouch that can offer a satisficing anal function in > 90% of patients with a good quality of life. This approach could be considered more aggressive, but it has surely determined a decrease in rate of patients needing surgery in emergency settings, consequently leading to lower incidence of perioperatory mortality and morbidity. However some aspects still need to be analyzed in order to offer better functional results, with lower complication rates, such as ideal pouch shape, type of pouch-anal anastomosis, the need for mucosectomy, the role of ileostomy, and, of course, a better understanding of physio-pathological mechanisms determining pouchitis is needed, even if such complication does not seem to affect significantly overall functional results.

7. References

Bartram, C.I. (1994) Plain abdominal x-ray in acute colitis. *Procededings of the Royal Society of Medicine* 69: 617-618

Bernstein, C.N.; Shanahan, F. & Weinstein, W.M. (1994) Are we telling patients the truth about surveillance colonoscopy in ulcerative colitis? *Lancet* 343: 71-74

Binder, V.; Both, H.; Hansen, P.K.; Hendriksen, C.; Kreiner, S. & Trop-Pedersen, K. (1982) Incidence and prevalence of Ulcerative Colitis and Crohn's disease in the country of Copenaghen 1962-1978. *Gastroenterology.* 83:563-568

Collins, R.H. Jr; Feldman, M. & Fordtran, J.S. (1987) Colon cancer, dysplasia, and surveillance in patients with ulcerative colitis. A critical review. *N Engl J Med* 316: 1654-1658

Connell, W.R. ; Talbot, I.C. ; Harpaz, N. ; Britto, N. ; Wilkinson, K.H. ; Kamm, M.A. & Lennard-Jones, J.E. (1994) Clinicopathological characteristics of colorectal carcinoma complicating ulcerative colitis. *Gut* 35: 1419-1423

Corbett, R.S. (1952) Recent advances in the surgical treatment of chronic ulcerative colitis. *Ann R Coll Surg Engl.* 10: 21-32

Devine, H. (1943) A method of colectomy for desperate cases of ulcerative colitis. *Surg Gynecol Obstet* 76: 136-138

Druss, R.G.; O'Connor, J.F.; Prudden, J.F. & Stern, O. (1968) Psychologic response to colectomy. *Arc Gen Psychiatry* 18: 53-59

Edwards, F.C. & Truelove, S.C. (1963) The course and prognosis of ulcerative colitis : Parts I and II : short-term and long-term prognosis. *Gut* 4:299-315

Farnell, M.B. & Adson, M.A. (1985) Ileorectostomy: current results: the Mayo Clinic Experience.. In: *Dozois RR (ed): Alternatives to Conventional Ileostomy. Year Book Medical Publisher*, Chicago, 100-121

Gyde, S.N.; Prior, P.; Allan, R.N.; Stevens, A.; Jewell, D.P.; Truelove, S.C.; Lofberg, R.; Brostrom, O. & Hellers, G (1988) Colorectal cancer in ulcerative colitis: a cohort study of primary referrals from three centres. *Gut* 29: 206-217

Hosie, H.B.; Grobler, S.P. & Keighley, M.R.B. (1992) Temporary loop ileostomy following restorative proctocolectomy. *Br J Surg.* 79: 33-34

Hyman, N.H.; Fazio, V.W. & Lavery, I.C. (1991) Consequence of ileal pouch anal anastomosis for Crohn's colitis. *Dis Colon Rectum.* 34 :653

Jewell, D.P. (1987) Ulcerative colitis.: indication for surgery. In: surgery of inflammatory bowel disorders. *Lee ECG, Ed. Edinburgh. Churchill Livingstone*, 33-38

Jones, P.F.; Munro, A. & Even, S.W.B. (1977) Colectomy and ileorectal anastomosis for colitis: report on a personal series with a critical review. *Br J Surg* 64: 615-623

Keighely, M.R.B.; Yoshioka, K. & Kmniot, W.A. (1991) Prospective randomized trial comparing anal function after hand sewn ileoanal anastomosis with mucosectomy versus stapled ileoanal anastomosis without mucosectomy in restorative proctocolectomy. *Br J Surg.* 78:430-434

Khubchandani, I.T.; Turinvei, H.D.; Sheets, J.A.; Stasik, J.J. & Kleckner, F.S. (1978) Ileorectal anastomosis for ulcerative and Crohn's colitis. *Am J Surg* 135: 751-756

Kirsner, J.B. & Shorter, R.G. (1982) Recent developments in "non specific" inflammatory bowel disease, Part I. *N Engl J Med* 306: 775-785

Kirsner, J.B. & Shorter, R.G. (1982) Recent developments in "non specific" inflammatory bowel disease, Part II. *N Engl J Med* 306: 837-848

Lavery, I.C.; Sirimarco, M.T.; Ziu, Y. & Fazio, V.W. Anal canal inflammation after ileal pouch-anal anastomosis. The need for treatment. *Dis Colon Rectum* 38:803-806

Leijonmarck, C.E.; Persson, P.G. & Hellers, G. (1990) Factors affecting colectomy rate in ulcerative colitis: an epidemiological study. *Gut* 31: 329-333

Lennard-Jones, J.E.; Ritchie, J.K.; Hilder, W. & Spicer, C.C. (1975) Assessment of severity in colitis. A preliminary study. *Gut* 579-84

Little, J.C. & Parks, A.G. (1977) Intersphincteric excision of the rectum. *Br J Surg* 64: 413-416

Lohmuller, J.L.; Pemberton, J.H. & Dozois P.R. (1990) Pouchitis and extraintestinal manifestations of inflammatory bowel disease after ileal pouch-anal anastomosis. *Ann Surg.* 21: 622-629

Marcello, P.W. (1993) Long-term results of the ileo-anal pouch procedure. *Arch Surg.* 128: 500-504

Metcalf, A.M.; Dozois, R.R. & Beart, R.W. (1988) Temporary ileostomy for pouch anal anastomosis . function and complication. *Dis Colon Rectum.* 29: 300-303

Mitchell, A.; Guyatt, G. & Singer, J. (1988) Quality of life in patients with inflammatory bowel disease. *J Clin Gastroenterol* 10: 306-310

Morson, B.C. (1962) Some peculiarities in the histology of intestinal polyps. *Dis Colon Rectum* 5: 337

Morson, B.C. & Pang, L.S.C. (1967) Rectal biopsy as aid to cancer control in ulcerative colitis. *Gut* 8: 423

Nicholls, R.J. (1993) Controversies and pratical problem solving. In : *Restorative Proctocolectomy*. Nicholls RJ, Bartolo DCC, Mortensen RJ. Oxford. Blackwell Scientific Publ, 53-82

Nicholls, R.J. & Pezim, M.E. (1984) Restorative proctocolectomy with ileal reservoir for ulcerative colitis and familial adenomatous polyposis. *Ann Surg* 199: 383-388

Nicholls, R.J. & Pezim, M.E. (1985) Restorative proctocolectomy with ileal reservoir for ulcerative colitis and familial adenomatous polyposis: a comparative of three reservoir designs. *Br J Surg* 72: 470-474

Parc, R.; Legrand, M. & Frileux, P. (1989) Comparative clinical results of ileal pouch-anal anastomosis and ileal ileorectal anastomosis in ulcerative colitis. *Hepatogastroenterology* 36: 235-239

Parker, M.C. & Nicholls, R.J. (1991) Restorative proctocolectomy in patients after previous intestinal or anal surgery. *Dis Colon Rectum* 35: 681

Parks, A.G. & Nicholls, R.J. (1978) Proctocolectomy without ileostomy for ulcerative colitis. *Br Med J* 2: 85-88

Patel, R.Y.; Barin, I.; Young, D. & Keighley, M.R.B. (1995) Cytokine production in pouchitis is similar to that in ulcerative colitis. *Dis Colon Rectum.* 38: 831-837

Pemberton, J.H.; Kelly, K.A.; Beart, R.W. Jr.; Dozois, R.R.; Wolff, B.G. & Ilstrup, D.M. (1987) Ileal pouch-anal anastomosis for chronic ulcerative colitis. Long term results. *Ann Surg* 206: 504-513

Pemberton, J.H. ; Kelly, K. ; Beart R.W. ; Dozois, R.R. ; Wolf, B.G. & Ilstrupp D.M. (1988) Ileal pouch anal anastomosis for chronic ulcerative colitis. *Ann Surg.* 207 : 504

Provenzale, D.; Kowdley, K.V.; Arora, S. & Wong, J.B. (1995) Prophylactic colectomy or surveillance for chronic ulcerative colitis? A decision analysis. *Gastroenterology* 109: 1188-1196

Richie, J. (1974) Results of surgery for inflammatory bowel disease: a furter study of one hospital region. *Br J Surg* 1:264-268

Romano, M.; Cuomo, A. ; Tuccillo, C.; Salerno, R.; Rocco, A.; Staibano, S.; Mascolo, M.; Sciaudone, G.; Mucherino, C.; Giuliani, A.; Riegler, G.; Nardone, G.; Del Vecchio Blanco, C. & Selvaggi, F. (2007) Vascular endothelial growth factor and cyclooxygenase-2 are overexpressed in ileal pouch-anal anastomosis. *Dis Colon Rectum* 50 (5):650-9

Sagar, P.M.; Lewis, W.; Holdsworth, P.J.; Johnston, D.; Mitchell, C. & MacFie, J. (1993) Quality of life after restorative proctocolectomy with a pelvic pouch compares favourably with that of patients with medically treated colitis. *Dis Colon Rectum.* 36: 584-592

Selvaggi, F.; Giuliani, A.; Gallo, C.; Signoriello, G.; Riegler, G. & Canonico, S. (2000) Randomized, controlled trial to compare the J-pouch and W-pouch configurations for ulcerative colitis in the maturation period. *Dis Colon Rectum* 43:615-620

Selvaggi, F.; Giuliani, A. & Sciaudone, G (2002) Le disfunzioni delle pouch ileali. *Archivio ed Atti della Soc.Ital. Chir.* 3: 144-160

Selvaggi, F.; Sciaudone, G.; Guadagni, I. & Pellino, G. (2010a) Ileal pouch-anal anastomosis after stapled haemorrhoidopexy for unrecognized ulcerative colitis. *Colorectal Dis.* 12:e172

Selvaggi, F.; Sciaudone, G.; Limongelli, P.; Di Stazio, C.; Guadagni, I.; Pellino, G.; De Rosa, M. & Riegler, G. (2010b) The effect of pelvic septic complications on function and quality of life after ileal pouch-anal anastomosis: a single center experience. *Am Surg.* 76:428-435

Selvaggi, F.; Silvestri, A.; Scotto Di Carlo, E. & Sciaudone, G (1996) Il trattamento chirurgico della rettocolite ulcerosa. *Tecniques in Coloproctol.* 4: 98-101

Skarsgard, E.D.; Atkinson, K.G.; Bell, G.A.; Pezim, M.E.; Seal, A.M. & Sharo, F.R. (1989) Function and quality of life results after ileal pouch surgery for chronic ulcerative colitis and for polyposis. *Am J Surg* 157: 457-471

Stonnington, C.M.; Phillips, S.F.; Melton, L.J. & Zinsmeister, A.R. (1987) Chronic ulcerative colitis: incidence and prevalence in a community. *Gut* 28: 402-409

Taylor, B.A.; Pemberton, J.H.; Carpenter, H.A.; Levin, K.E.; Schroeder, K.W.; Welling, D.R.; Spencer, M.P. & Zinsmeister, A.R. (1992) Dysplasia in chronic ulcerative colitis: implications for colonoscopic surveillance. *Dis Colon Rectum* 35: 950-956

Truelove, S.C. (1988) Medical management of ulcerative colitis and indication for colectomy. *Worl J Surg.* 12: 142-147

Truelove, S.C. & Jewell, D.P. (1974) Intensive intravenous regimen for severe attack of ulcerative colitis. *Lancet* i: 1067-1074

Truelove, S.C. & Witts, L.J. (1955) Cortisone in ulcerative colitis: final report on a therapeutic trial. *Br Med J* 2:1041-1048

Turnbull, R.B.; Hawk, W.A. & Weakly, F.I. (1971) Surgical treatment of toxic megacolon: ileostomy and colostomy to prepare patients for colectomy. *Am J Surg* 122: 325-331

Utsonomiya, A.J.; Iwama, T.; Iamjo, M.; Matsuo, S.; Sawai, S.; Yalgashi, K. & Hirayama, R. (1980) Total Colectomy, mucosal proctectomy and ileoanal anastomosis. *Dis Colon Rectum* 23: 459-466

van Heerden, J.A. & Beart, R.W. Jr (1980) Carcinoma of the colon and rectum complicating chronic ulcerative colitis. *Dis Colon Rectum* 23: 155-159

Williams, N.S. (1989) Restorative proctocolectomy is the first choice elective surgical treatment for ulcerative colitis. *Br J Surg* 76: 1109

Williams, N.S. & Johnston, D (1985) The current state of mucosal proctectomy and ileo-anal anastomosis in the surgical treatment of ulcerative colitis and familial polyposis. *Br J Surg.* 72: 159-168

Ziv, Y.; Fazio, V.W.; Church, J.M.; Milsom, J.W. & Schroeder, T.K. (1995) Safety of urgent restorative proctocolectomy with ileal pouch-anal anastomosis for fulminant colitis. *Dis Colon Rectum*, 38: 345-349

2

Laparoscopic Surgery for Severe Ulcerative Colitis

Kazuhiro Watanabe, Hitoshi Ogawa, Chikashi Shibata, Koh Miura, Takeshi Naitoh, Masayuki Kakyou, Takanori Morikawa, Sho Haneda, Naoki Tanaka, Katsuyoshi Kudo, Shinobu Ohnuma, Hiyroyuki Sasaki and Iwao Sasaki
Department of Surgery, Tohoku University Graduate School of Medicine
Japan

1. Introduction

Ulcerative colitis is occasionally exacerbated by fulminant manifestation of colitis. Severe ulcerative colitis is usually defined based on Trulove and Witts' criteria (Table 1) (Truelove & Witts, 1955). The incidence of severe colitis in ulcerative colitis is 5 to 15 percent (Chen et al., 1998). If the patient is not improving despite intensive medical therapy, emergency colectomy is mandatory. In such a case, the patient is often malnourished and anemic, and has received high dose of steroids; therefore, the usual option in patients with severe ulcerative colitis is subtotal colectomy and ileostomy with preservation of the rectum (Gurland & Wexner, 2002). Restorative proctectomy can be done at a later time after the patient has recovered fully and steroids have been withdrawn (Fig. 1).

(1) >6 stools/day
(2) Bloody diarrhea
(3) Fever ≥37.5°C
(4) Heart rate ≥90/ min
(5) Hemoglobin ≤10g/dl
(6) Erythrocyte sedimentation rate ≥30mm/hr

Table 1. Definition of severe ulcerative colitis based on Trulove and Witts' criteria (Truelove & Witts, 1955). When criteria (1) and (2) are applied, either criterion (3) or (4) is applied, and four of the six criteria are applied, the ulcerative colitis is diagnosed as severe

The earliest reports of the laparoscopic approach to ulcerative colitis in the elective setting are from the early 1990s (Peters, 1992; Wexner et al., 1992). These first results did not seem very promising, the laparoscopic technique appeared too difficult to apply, too time-consuming, and comorbidity was high. The authors discouraged the use of laparoscopic approach for patients requiring total colectomy. However, with advances in technology and experience of laparoscopic surgery, more favourable results have been stated (Marcello et al., 2000; Brown et al., 2001; Hamel et al., 2001; Hashimoto et al., 2001; Seshadri et al., 2001; Ky et al., 2002; Gill et al., 2004; Kienle et al., 2005; Larson et al., 2005). These reports have shown the advantages of laparoscopic total colectomy such as reduced postoperative pain, earlier return of intestinal function, decreased length of hospital stay, and improved cosmesis (Table 2). On the basis of these results, recent studies have evaluated the feasibility and safety of minimally invasive surgery for selected patients with severe ulcerative colitis. Minimally invasive surgery techniques include laparoscopic-assisted colectomy and hand-assisted laparoscopic surgery. In this article, an overview of current status of minimally invasive surgery to severe ulcerative colitis is provided.

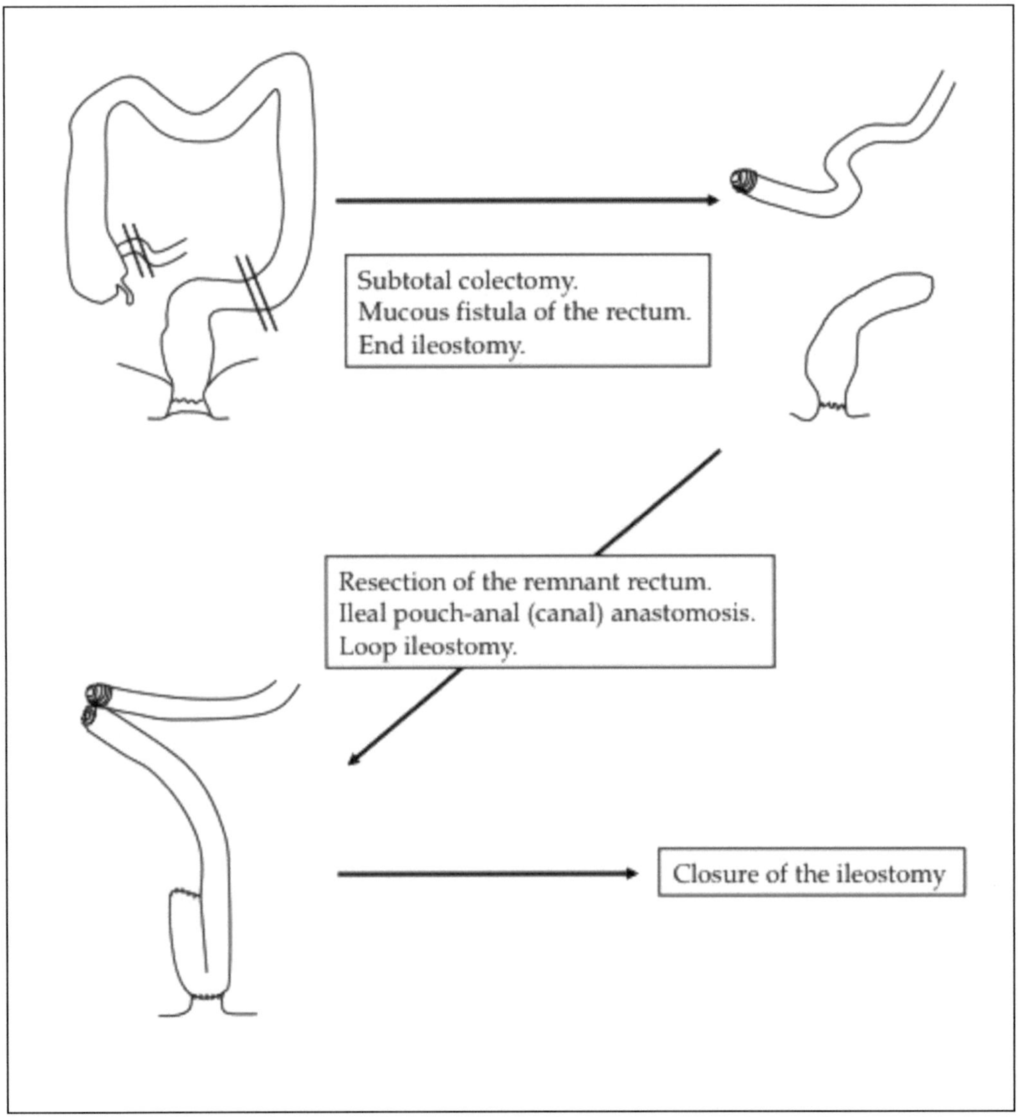

Fig. 1. Three-stage restorative proctocolectomy for severe ulcerative colitis

Author (year)	Number of patients		Operative time (min)			Conversion (%)
	Lap	Open	Lap	Open	*P*-value	Lap
Marcello (2000)	20 (UC;13 FAP;7)	20 (UC;13 FAP;7)	330	225	<0.001	0
Hashimoto (2001)	11 (UC;6 FAP;5)	13 (UC;6 FAP;7)	483	402	<0.05	0
Gill (2004)	14 (UC;13 FAP;1)	-	260	-	-	7
Kienle (2005)	50 (UC;23 FAP;27)	-	320	-	-	8
Larson (2005)	33 (UC;31 FAP;2)	33 (UC;31 FAP;2)	-	-	-	-

UC: ulcerative colitis, FAP: familial ademnomatous polyposis

Table 2. Perioperative data from clinical trials treating laparoscopic-assisted restorative proctocolectomy and ileo-anal anastomosis in elective setting

Author	Hospital stay (days)			Morbidity (%)		
	Lap	Open	*P*-value	Lap	Open	*P*-value
Marcello	7	8	0.02	20	25	NS
Hashimoto	24.1	31.3	<0.05	55	38	0.453
Gill	7	-	-	29	-	-
Kienle	12	-	-	30	-	-
Larson	-	-	-	6	12	0.39

Table 2 (continued). Perioperative data from clinical trials treating laparoscopic-assisted restorative proctocolectomy and ileo-anal anastomosis in elective setting

Author	Conclusion
Marcello	Technically feasible and safe. Shorter hospital stay. Quicker return of bowel function. Complication rates were similar to open surgery.
Hashimoto	Better cosmetic results. Reduce the degree of postoperative pain. Shorter hospital stay.
Gill	Technically feasible. Operative time was acceptable.
Kienle	Technically feasible. LAP may reduce the need for perioperative blood transfusion.
Larson	The function and quality of life outcomes seemed to be equivalent to open surgery.

Table 2 (continued). Perioperative data from clinical trials treating laparoscopic-assisted restorative proctocolectomy and ileo-anal anastomosis in elective setting

2. Indication for minimally invasive surgery in severe ulcerative colitis

Patients are usually hospitalized and received intensive medical therapy when their severe colitis is diagnosed. The mainstay of treatment for severe ulcerative colitis is Truelove's intensive intravenous steroid regimen (Truelove & Jewell 1974). Immunosuppressive therapy, cytapheresis therapy, and/or steroid pulse therapy are considered as alternative treatment options (Lichtiger et al., 1994; Sawada et al., 1995; Sood et al., 2002). Total parenteral nutrition, albumin and blood transfusion, and/or antibiotic therapy are considered as supportive therapies. Surgery is indicated when the patients are unresponsive to medical therapy, or when massive hemorrhage, toxic megacolon, or perforation occurs. Patients with severe ulcerative colitis are often malnourished and anemic, and has received high dose of steroids, which increase the likelihood of postoperative complications.

Minimally invasive surgery for severe ulcerative colitis is technically difficult because of active inflammation and induration of the mesentery, fragile intestinal tissue, abscesses between intestinal loops, and dense adhesions. To date, there is no randomized controlled trial assessing minimally invasive surgery for severe ulcerative colitis. In most retrospective studies, the patients with complications such as toxic megacolon, intestinal perforation, peritonitis, or shock stage were excluded from the indication for minimally invasive surgery (Table 3).

(1) Toxic megacolon
(2) Intestinal perforation
(3) Peritonitis
(4) Shock status

Table 3. Exclusion criteria for minimally invasive surgery in severe ulcerative colitis

3. Laparoscopic-assisted subtotal colectomy for severe ulcerative colitis

Several recent studies have reported the outcome of laparoscopic-assisted subtotal colectomy in selected patients with severe ulcerative colitis (Table 4). In most of these studies, patients with complications such as toxic megacolon, intestinal perforation, peritonitis, or shock status were excluded from the indication for minimally invasive surgery.

Author (year)	Number of patients		Operative time (min)			Conversion (%)
	Lap	Open	Lap	Open	*P*-value	Lap
Telem (2010)	29	61	216	170	<0.01	7
Maggiori (2010)	35 (UC;27 CD;8)	-	252	-	-	6
Fowkes (2008)	32	-	135	-	-	3
Maeceau (2007)	40 (UC;26CD;13 IC;1)	48 (UC;14 CD;29 IC;5)	253	231	NS	5
Bell (2002)	18	6	220 ~ 360	-	-	0
Dunker (2000)	10 (UC;8 CD;2)	22 (UC;27 CD;5)	271	150	<0.001	0

UC: ulcerative colitis, FAP: familial ademnomatous polyposis

Table 4. Perioperative data from clinical trials treating laparoscopic-assisted subtotal colectomy for severe ulcerative colitis

Telem *et al* (Telem et al., 2010) from the Mount Sinai Medical Center, New York City evaluated laparoscopic-assisted subtotal colectomy (n=29) versus open subtotal colectomy (n=61) in patients with ulcerative colitis requiring urgent or emergent operative intervention. Two (7%) patients in the laparoscopic group required conversion to open surgery. The mean operative time was significantly longer in the laparoscopic group (216.4 vs. 169.9 min, $P<0.01$). Intraoperative blood loss was significantly lower in the laparoscopic group (130.4 vs. 201.4 ml, $p<0.05$). The mean hospital stay was shorter in laparoscopic group (4.53 vs. 6 days, $p<0.001$). The rate of wound complication was significantly lower in laparoscopic group (0 vs. 21 percent, $p<0.01$).

Maggiori *et al* (Maggiori et al., 2010) from Beaujon Hospital, France evaluated the outcome of laparoscopic-assisted subtotal colectomy with double end ileo-sigmoidostomy in patients with acute or severe colitis. The medical records of 35 patients (Ulcerative colitis, n=27; Crohn's disease, n=8) were reviewed. Two (6%) patients required conversion to open surgery because of intra-abdominal adhesions (n=1), and complicated case with perforated acute colitis (n=1). The mean operative time was 252 minutes. The mean hospital stay was 8 days. Five (15%) patients experienced postoperative complications and no reoperation was needed. With a mean delay of 80 ± 20 days (range: 43 to 129 days), intestinal continuity was restored in 100 percent of the cases.

Fowkes *et al* (Fowkes et al., 2008) from Frenchay Hospital, United Kingdom analyzed surgical outcomes of fulminate and medically resistant ulcerative colitis carried out laparoscopically. The medical records of 32 patients were reviewed. One (3%) patient required conversion to open surgery because of a small, localized perforation (unsuspected preoperatively). The median operative time was 135 minutes. The median hospital stay was 8 days. Twelve (38%) patients experienced postoperative complications. They concluded that laparoscopic-assisted subtotal colectomy in fulminant and medically resistant ulcerative colitis was feasible, safe and largely predictable operations that allow for early hospital discharge.

Author (year)	Hospital stay (days)			Morbidity (%)		
	Lap	Open	*P*-value	Lap	Open	*P*-value
Telem (2010)	4.5	6	<0.001	28 Wound complication 0	34 Wound complication 21	NS <0.01
Maggiori (2010)	8	-	-	15	-	-
Fowkes (2008)	8	-	-	38	-	-
Maeceau (2007)	9	12	NS (<0.10)	35	56	NS (<0.10)
Bell (2002)	5.1	8.8	<0.05	33	-	-
Dunker (2000)	14.6	18.0	0.05	Minor complication 10 Major complication 30	Minor complication2 5 Major complication2 8	0.41 1.00

Table 4 (continued). Perioperative data from clinical trials treating laparoscopic-assisted subtotal colectomy for severe ulcerative colitis

Marceau *et al* (Marceau et al., 2007) from Beaujon Hospital, France conducted a case-matched study to assess the feasibility and safety of laparoscopic-assisted subtotal colectomy (*n*=40) (Ulcerative colitis, n=14; Crohn's disease, n=29; Indeterminate colitis, n=5) compared with open subtotal colectomy (*n*=48) (Ulcerative colitis, n=26; Crohn's disease, n=13; Indeterminate colitis, n=1) in patients with severe colitis. Two (5%) patients required conversion to open surgery because of intensive adhesions (*n*=1) and colonic fistula (*n*=1). Between the laparoscopic group and open group, the mean operative time (253 vs. 231 min), overall morbidity (35 vs. 56%), and hospital stay (9 vs. 12 days) were similar. After a follow-up of 3 ± 4 months after the first operation, 35 patients (88%) have had restorative intestinal continuity through laparoscopic approach or elective incision at the site of previous stoma. They concluded that laparoscopic-assisted subtotal colectomy was as safe and effective as open subtotal colectomy for patients with severe colitis complicating inflammatory bowel disease.

Bell *et al* (Bell & Seymour 2002) from Yale University School of Medicine, New Haven reported surgical outcomes of fulminant ulcerative colitis carried out laparoscopically. The medical records of 18 patients with poorly controlled fulminant ulcerative colitis on aggressive immunosuppressive therapy who underwent laparoscopic subtotal colectomy were reviewed. None of the laparoscopic procedures required conversion to an open operation, and there were no intraoperative complications. The total operative time ranged from 220 to 360 min. Procedure length diminished significantly over the course of the series; the operative time during the last six procedures was 244 vs. 275 minutes during the prior 12 patients. Postoperative hospital stay was 5.0 days vs. 8.8 days (p<0.05) for a group of 6 patients who had undergone open subtotal colectomy for the same indications. Postoperative complications occurred in 6 (33%) patients.

Author (year)	Conclusions
Telem (2010)	Technically feasible and safe. Improved cosmesis. Reduced intraoperative blood loss. Negligible wound complications. Shorter hospital stay.
Maggiori (2010)	Low morbidity. Facilitated second step of intestinal continuity restoration for both ileorectal and ileo-anal anastomosis.
Fowkes (2008)	Technically feasible and safe. Shorter hospital stay. Facilitated subsequent proctectomy and pouch construction.
Marceau (2007)	Operative time, overall morbidity, and hospital stay were similar to open surgery. 84% of the patients underwent restorative intestinal continuity
Bell (2002)	Technically feasible. Shorter hospital stay. Facilitated subsequent proctectomy and pouch construction.
Dunker (2000)	Technically feasible and safe. Shorter hospital stay. Longer operative time.

Table 4 (continued). Perioperative data from clinical trials treating laparoscopic-assisted subtotal colectomy for severe ulcerative colitis

Dunker et al (Dunker et al., 2000) from Academic Medical Center, Netherlands evaluated the feasibility and safety of emergency laparoscopic-assisted subtotal colectomy in patients with severe acute colitis. The medical records of 42 consecutive patients (Laparoscopic group; n=10, Open group; n=32) were reviewed. No patients in laparoscopic group required conversion to open surgery. The mean operative time was longer in laparoscopic group than in the open group (271 vs. 150 minutes). Postoperative hospital stay was significantly shorter in the laparoscopic group than in the open group (14.6 vs. 18.0 days. Complications were similar for the two groups. They concluded that laparoscopic-assisted subtotal colectomy in patients with severe acute colitis was feasible and safe as open colectomy.

4. Hand-assisted laparoscopic subtotal colectomy for severe ulcerative colitis

Standard laparoscopic assisted subtotal colectomy for severe ulcerative colitis is still technically difficult because of bowel friability and hypervascularity, creating a high likelihood of perforation and bleeding. Hand-assisted laparoscopic surgery is a technique in which laparoscopic procedures are performed with the aid of a hand inserted into the abdomen through a small incision. (Ballantyne & Leahy, 2004; Nakajima et al., 2004; Rivadeneira et al., 2004; Boushey et al., 2007). Surgeons are abled to obtain tactile sensation, manual retraction, and digital vascular control, which could allow complex laparoscopic operations to be performed more effectively and satisfactorily. A few recent studies have reported hand-assisted laparoscopic subtotal colectomy for selected patients with severe ulcerative colitis (Watanabe et al., 2009; Holubar et al., 2009; Chung et al., 2009).

4.1 Surgical technique for hand-assisted laparoscopic subtotal colectomy

The patient was placed in the supine position with legs moderately opened. A 70-mm lower paramedian incision was made and the abdomen was entered (Fig. 2). The ascending and descending colon was manually mobilized through the incision. After the mobilization, the hand port was placed in the lower paramedian incision. A 12-mm trocar was inserted above the umbilicus for laparoscope and pneumoperitoneum. A 5-mm or 12-mm trocar was inserted in the lower left abdomen for dissection. If necessary, the third 5-mm or 12-mm trocar was inserted in the upper left abdomen. The greater omentum was dissected and splenocolic and hepatocolic ligaments were taken down to mobilize the transverse colon by use of a Harmonic Scalpel™ (UltraCision, Smithfield, RI) or LigaSure™ (Tyco Healthcare Japan, Tokyo, Japan) (Fig.3, 4). The mesocolon was also dissected. The ileocolic artery was preserved in all patients to provide optimal blood supply to the distal ileum. After this, the laparoscopic procedure was ended. Transsection of the terminal ileum and proximal rectum were performed with a linear stapler, and the colon was taken out through the lower paramedian incision. A mucous fistula of the rectum was constructed in the left lower abdomen, and a standard Brooke ileostomy was fashioned in the right lower abdomen (Fig. 5).

4.2 Hand-assisted laparoscopic surgery for severe ulcerative colitis

A few recent studies have evaluated the outcome of hand-assisted laparoscopic subtotal colectomy in patients with severe ulcerative colitis.

The authors (Watanabe et al., 2009) from Tohoku University Graduate School of Medicine, Japan recently reviewed the medical records of 60 patients who underwent emergency subtotal colectomy with hand-assisted laparoscopic technique (n=30) or conventional open technique (n=30) for severe ulcerative colitis. One (3%) patient in the laparoscopic group required conversion to open surgery because of excessive inflammatory adhesion. The median operative time was significantly longer in the hand-assisted laparoscopic surgery group than in the open surgery group (242 vs. 191 minutes; $P<0.001$). The median time to first solid diet in the hand-assisted laparoscopic surgery group was significantly shorter than that in the open surgery group (4.8 vs. 5.9 days; $P=0.007$). The postoperative hospital stay in the hand-assisted laparoscopic surgery group was significantly shorter than in the open surgery group (23.0 vs. 33.0 days; $P=0.001$). The number of postoperative complications during the hospital stay in the hand-assisted laparoscopic surgery group was significantly less than in open surgery group (37 vs. 63%; $P = 0.041$). Four (13%) patients in the open surgery group required relaparotomy because of peritoneal abscess (two patients) or strangulation ileus (two patients), but no patients needed relaparotomy in the hand-assisted laparoscopic surgery group ($P=0.040$). In the open surgery group, 4 of 30 patients (13%) had surgical site infection and 2 patients among them developed wound dehiscence

and needed resuture of the wound. In the hand-assisted surgery group, 4 of 30 patients (13%) had surgical site infection, but no patient developed wound dehiscence. The authors concluded that hand-assisted laparoscopic surgery can be an alternative to conventional open surgery for severe ulcerative colitis.
conversion to open surgery was 2 (5.5%) in laparoscopic-assisted surgery group, and 1 (7.1%) in hand-assisted laparoscopic surgery group, respectively. The median operative time was 251 minutes. The median hospital stay was 4 days. Seventeen (34%) patients experienced postoperative complications and 2 (4%) patients required reoperation. The most frequent complications after each procedure were ileus (8%) and surgical site infections (4%).

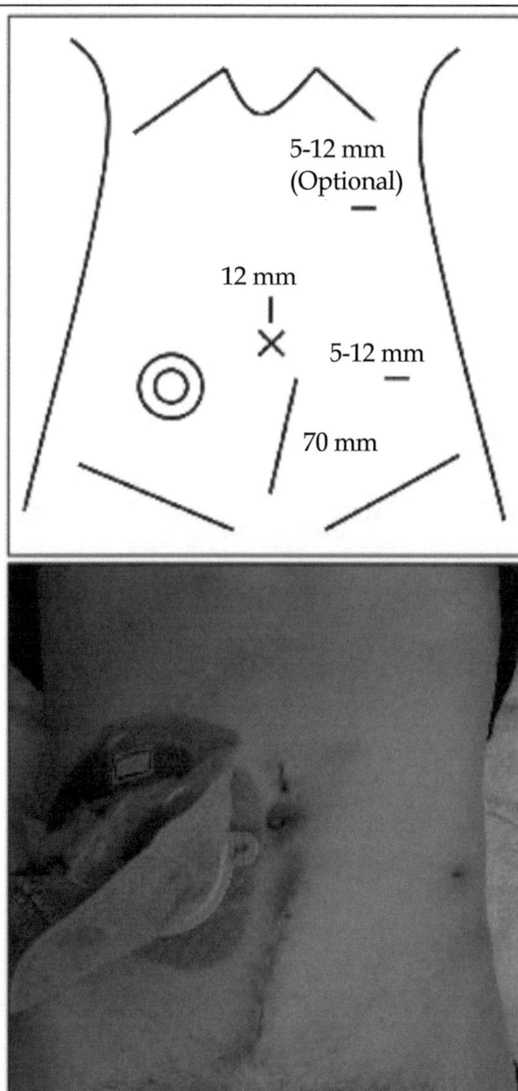

Fig. 2. Port and incision placement for hand-assisted laparoscopic subtotal colectomy (above). Operative scars after hand-assisted laparoscopic subtotal colectomy (below)

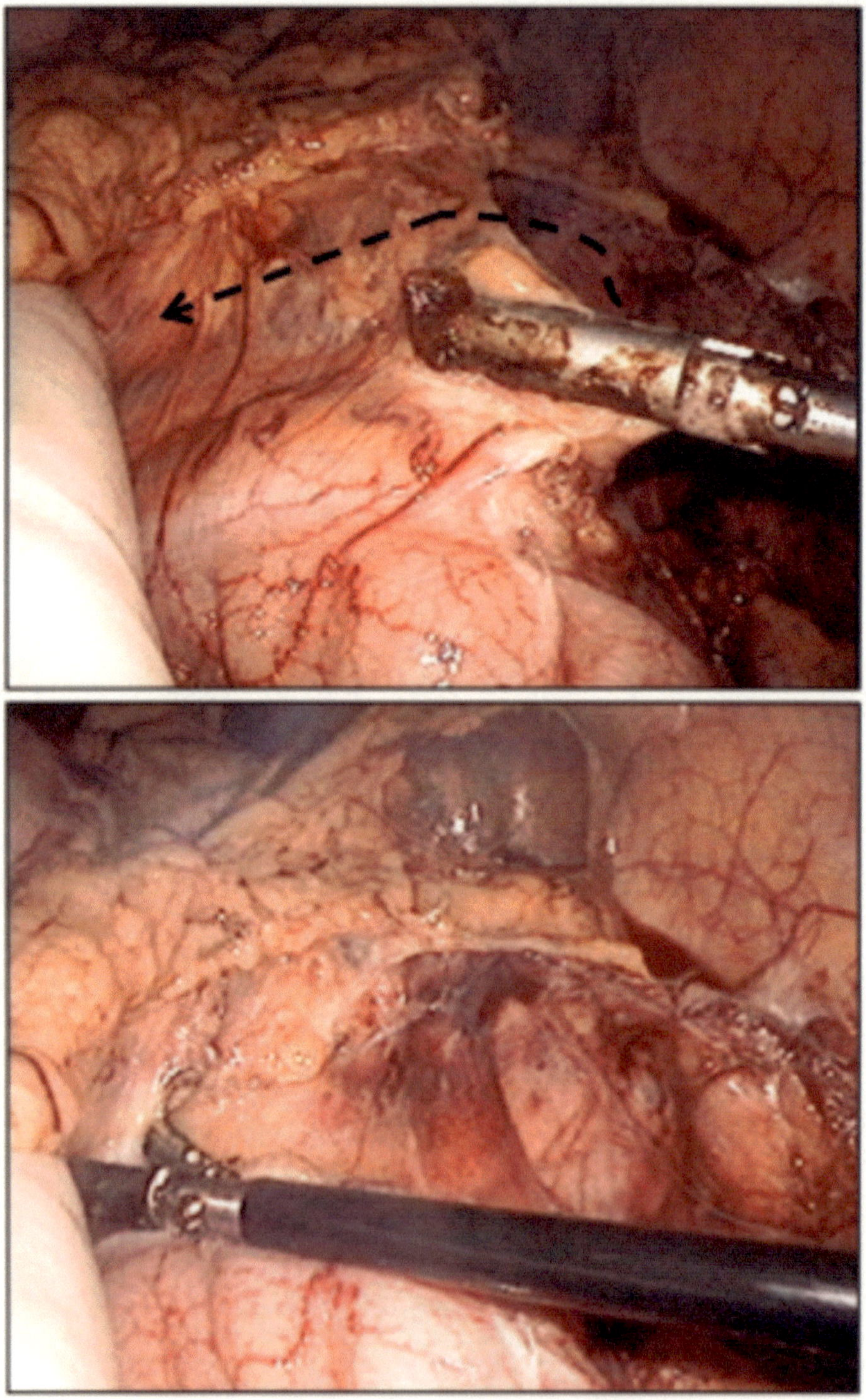

Fig. 3. Mobilization of the transverse colon using hand-assisted laparoscopic technique. Splenocolic ligament was taken down from the descending colon to the transverse colon

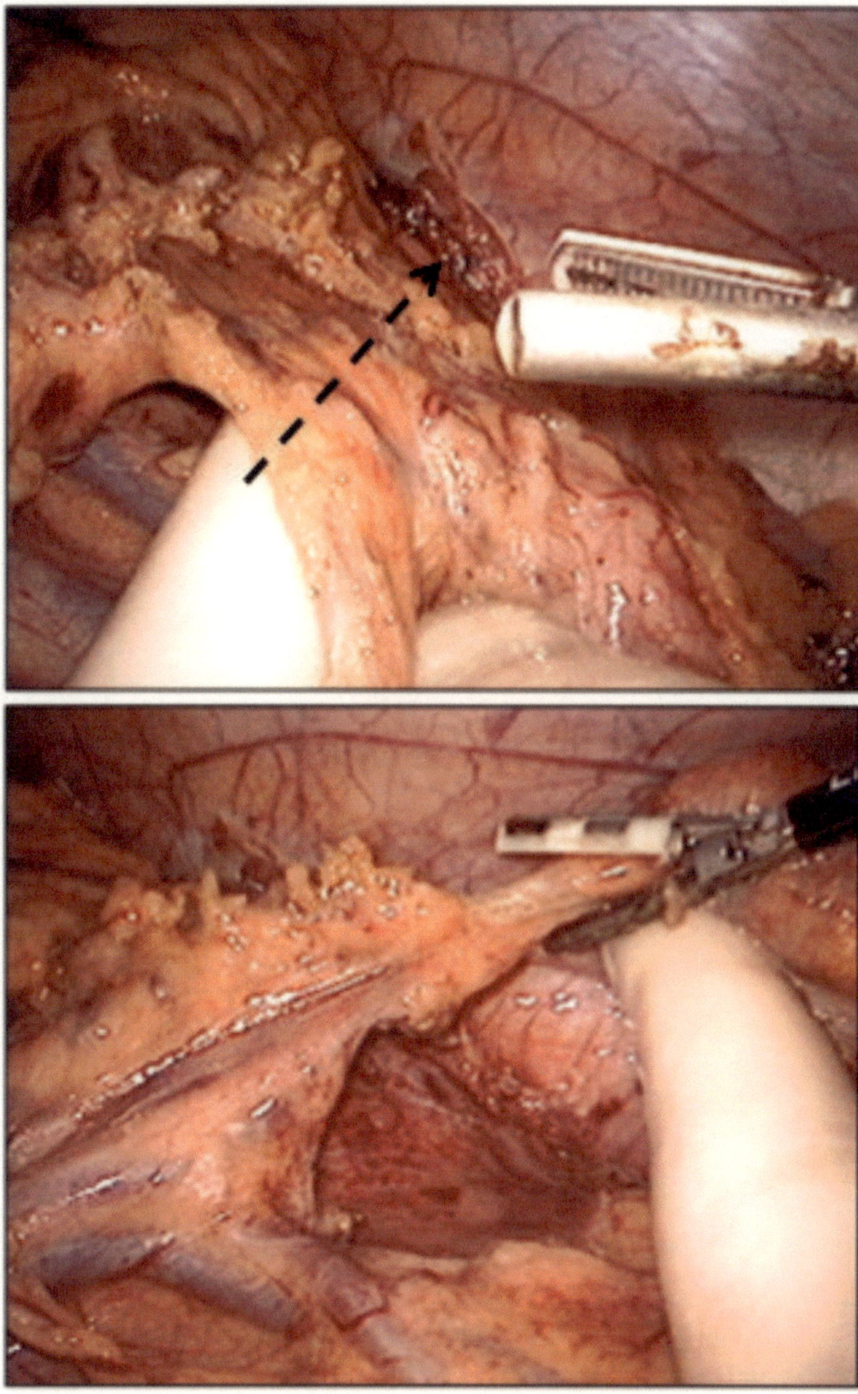

Fig. 4. Mobilization of the transverse colon using hand-assisted laparoscopic technique. Splenocolic ligament was taken down from the transverse colon to the descending colon

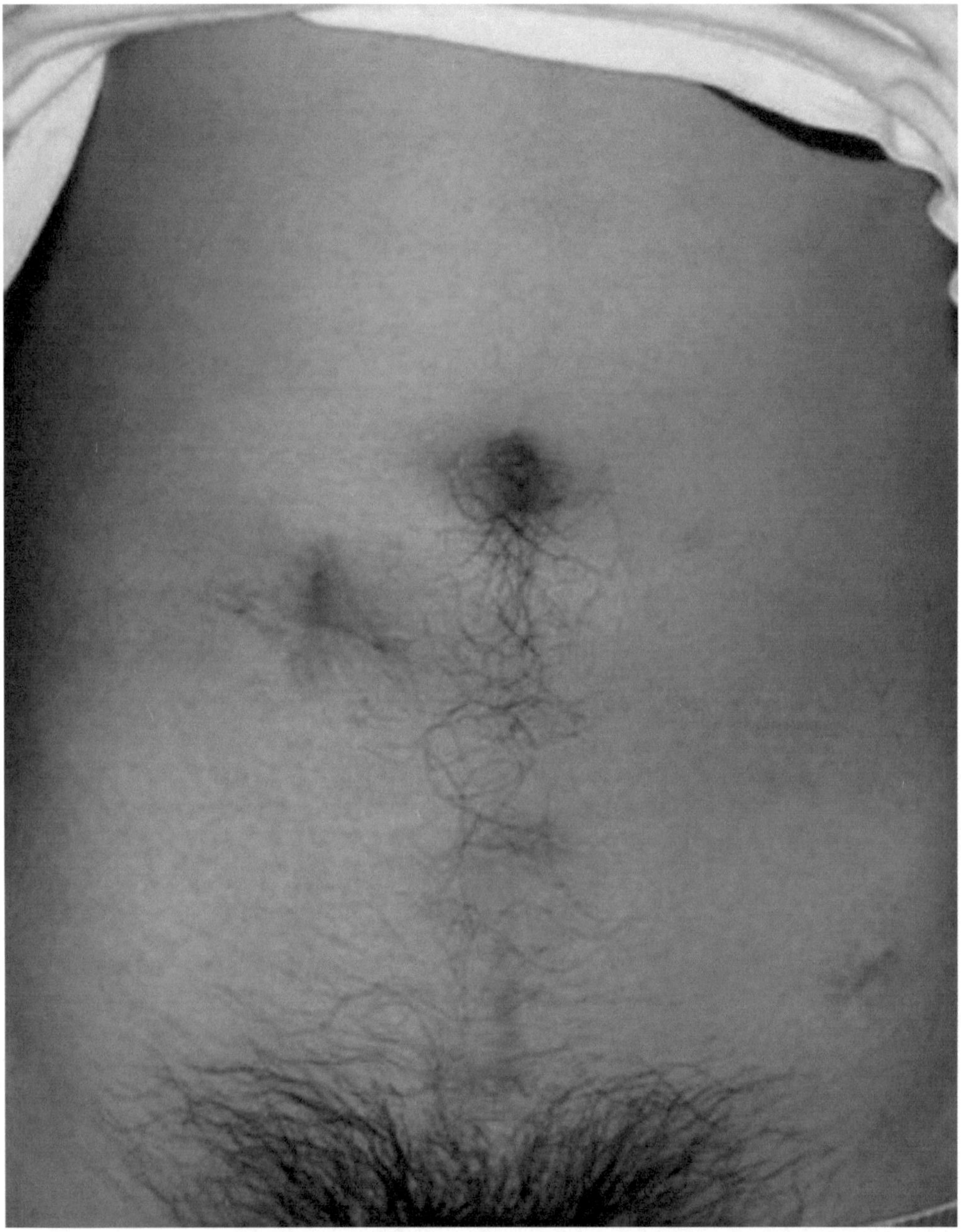

Fig. 5. Operative scars after three-stage hand-assisted laparoscopic proctocolectomy

Holubar *et al* (Holubar et al., 2009) from Mayo Clinic, Rochester evaluated the safety and feasibility of minimally invasive subtotal colectomy for fulminant ulcerative colitis. The medical records of 50 patients (Laparoscopic-assisted surgery; n=36, Hand-assisted laparoscopic surgery; n=14) were reviewed. The number of patients who required Chung *et al* (Chung et al., 2009) from Washington University School of Medicine, St. Louis compared short-term outcomes of minimally invasive vs. open subtotal colectomy for severe ulcerative colitis. The medical records of 81 patients (Laparoscopic-assisted surgery; *n*=17, Hand-assisted laparoscopic surgery; *n*=20, Open surgery; *n*=44) were reviewed. Two (11.8%) patients in minimally invasive surgery group required conversion to open surgery because of bleeding from the middle colic vessels, and colonic injury with feculent spillage. Intraoperative intravenous fluid volume, operative time, and estimated blood loss were increased in the minimally invasive surgery group. Short-term recovery (return of bowel function, length of stay, inpatient narcotic use, and complication rate) was significantly lessened in the minimally invasive surgery group. The minimally invasive surgery group completed all three stages a mean of 66 days sooner than the open surgery group (188.9 vs. 255.36 days, P = 0.0038).

Author (year)	Number of patients		Operative time (min)			Conversion (%)
	MIS	Open	MIS	Open	*P*-value	MIS
Watanabe (2009)	HALS;30	30	242	191	<0.001	3
Holubar (2009)	HALS;14 LAP;36	-	251	-	-	HALS;7.1 LAP;5.5
Chung (2009)	HALS;20 LAP;17	44	223	140	<0.001	Overall; 11.8

MIS: minimally invasive surgery

Table 5. Perioperative data from clinical trials treating laparoscopic-assisted subtotal colectomy for severe ulcerative colitis

Author (year)	Hospital stay (days)			Morbidity (%)		
	MIS	Open	*P*-value	MIS	Open	*P*-value
Watanabe (2009)	23	33	0.001	37	63	0.041
Holubar (2009)	4	-	-	34	-	-
Chung (2009)	4.9	8.5	0.039	24	48	0.039

MIS: minimally invasive surgery

Table 5 (Continued). Perioperative data from clinical trials treating laparoscopic-assisted subtotal colectomy for severe ulcerative colitis

Author (year)	Conclusions
Watanabe (2009)	Technically feasible and safe. Longer operative time. Shorter hospital stay. Reduced postoperative complication rate.
Holubar (2009)	Technically feasible and safe. Shorter hospital stay.
Chung (2009)	Safe. Associated with short-term benefits that may lead to faster recovery and progression to completion of restorative proctocolectomy.

Table 5 (continued). Perioperative data from clinical trials treating laparoscopic-assisted subtotal colectomy for severe ulcerative colitis

5. Conclusion

The earliest reports of the laparoscopic approach to ulcerative colitis in the elective setting provided little evidence of significant benefit over the standard open operative approach (Peters 1992; Wexner et al. 1992). However, with advances in technology and experience of laparoscopic surgery, more favourable results have been stated. Several studies have reported the feasibility and safety of laparoscopic assisted total colectomy for ulcerative colitis in the elective setting, and shown the advantages of laparoscopic assisted total colectomy such as reduced postoperative pain, earlier return of intestinal function, decreased length of hospital stay, and improved cosmesis (Marcello et al., 2000; Hashimoto et al., 2001; Seshadri et al., 2001; Gill et al., 2004; Kienle et al., 2005; Larson et al., 2005). On the basis of these results, several studies have evaluated the feasibility and safety of minimally invasive surgery for selected patients with severe ulcerative colitis (Dunker et al., 2000; Bell & Seymour, 2002; Marceau et al., 2007; Fowkes et al., 2008; Watanabe et al., 2009; Holubar et al., 2009; Chung et al., 2009; Maggiori et al., 2010; Telem et al., 2010). These retrospective trials indicated that minimally invasive subtotal colectomy for selected patients with severe ulcerative colitis associated with a marked reduction in wound complication rate, time to return of bowel function, and mean hospital stay, although most of these studies have reported that the mean operating time was longer than open surgery. The role of minimally invasive surgery for patients with severe ulcerative colitis is still not well defined because there is no randomized clinical trial; however, the reproducibility of the results among many institutions provides adequate evidence to demonstrate clear advantages of minimally invasive surgery for severe ulcerative colitis over a conventional open surgery. Laparoscopic assisted surgery for severe ulcerative colitis is still technically difficult because of bowel friability and hypervascularity, creating a high likelihood of perforation and bleeding. A few recent studies assessed hand-assisted laparoscopic surgery for selected patients with severe ulcerative colitis (Watanabe et al., 2009; Holubar et al., 2009; Chung et al., 2009). The use of this technique may be adequate for severe ulcerative colitis because hand-assisted surgery enables surgeons to obtain tactile sensation, manual retraction, and digital vascular control, which could allow complex laparoscopic operations to be performed more effectively and satisfactorily. Further evidence based study is needed to clarify the role of laparoscopic assisted or hand-assisted laparoscopic surgery for severe ulcerative colitis.

6. References

Ballantyne, G. H. & Leahy, P.F. (2004). Hand-assisted laparoscopic colectomy: evolution to a clinically useful technique. *Dis Colon Rectum* 47(5): 753-765.

Bell, R. L. & Seymour, N. E. (2002). Laparoscopic treatment of fulminant ulcerative colitis. *Surgical endoscopy* 16(12): 1778-1782.

Boushey, R. P, Marcello, P. W., Martel, G., Rusin, L. C., Roberts, P. L., & Schoetz, D. J., Jr. (2007). Laparoscopic total colectomy: an evolutionary experience. *Dis Colon Rectum* 50(10): 1512-1519.

Brown, S. R., Eu K. W., & Seow-Choen, F. (2001). Consecutive series of laparoscopic-assisted vs. minilaparotomy restorative proctocolectomies. *Dis Colon Rectum* 44(3): 397-400.

Chen, H. H., Wexner, S. D., Weiss, E. G., Nogueras, J. J., Alabaz, O., Iroatulam, A. J., Nessim, A., & Joo, J. S. (1998). Laparoscopic colectomy for benign colorectal disease is associated with a significant reduction in disability as compared with laparotomy. *Surg Endosc* 12(12): 1397-1400.

Chung, T.P., Fleshman, J.W., Birnbaum, E.H., Hunt, S.R., Dietz, D.W., Read, T.E., & Mutch, M.G., (2009). Laparoscopic vs. open total abdominal colectomy for severe colitis: impact on recovery and subsequent completion restorative proctectomy. *Dis Colon Rectum* 52(1): 4-10.

Dunker, M. S., Bemelman, W. A., Slors, J. F., van Hogezand, R. A., Ringers, J., & Gouma, D. J. (2000). Laparoscopic-assisted vs open colectomy for severe acute colitis in patients with inflammatory bowel disease (IBD): a retrospective study in 42 patients. *Surgical Endosc* 14(10): 911-914.

Fowkes, L., Krishna, K., Menon, A., Greenslade, G. L., & Dixon, A. R. (2008). Laparoscopic emergency and elective surgery for ulcerative colitis. *Colorectal disease* 10(4): 373-378.

Gill, T. S., Karantana, A., Rees, J., Pandey, S., & Dixon, A. R. (2004). Laparoscopic proctocolectomy with restorative ileal-anal pouch. *Colorectal disease* 6(6): 458-461.

Gurland, B. H., & Wexner, S. D. (2002). Laparoscopic surgery for inflammatory bowel disease: results of the past decade. *Inflammatory bowel diseases* 8(1): 46-54.

Hamel, C. T., Hildebrandt, U., Weiss, E. G., Feifelz, G., & Wexner, S. D. (2001). Laparoscopic surgery for inflammatory bowel disease. *Surg Endosc* 15(7): 642-645.

Hashimoto, A., Funayama, Y., Naito, H., Fukushima, K., Shibata, C., Naitoh, T., Shibuya, K., Koyama, K., Takahashi, K., Ogawa, H., Satoh, S., Ueno, T., Kitayama, T., Matsuno, S., & Sasaki, I. (2001). Laparascope-assisted versus conventional restorative proctocolectomy with rectal mucosectomy. *Surg Today* 31(3): 210-214.

Holubar, S. D., Larson, D. W., Dozois, E. J., Pattana-Arun, J., Pemberton, J. H., & Cima, R. R. (2009). Minimally invasive subtotal colectomy and ileal pouch-anal anastomosis for fulminant ulcerative colitis: a reasonable approach? *Dis Colon Rectum* 52(2): 187-192.

Kienle, P., Z'Graggen, K., Schmidt, J., Benner, A., Weitz, J., & Buchler, M. W. (2005). Laparoscopic restorative proctocolectomy. *Br J Surg* 92(1): 88-93.

Ky, A. J., Sonoda, T., & Milsom, J. W. (2002). One-stage laparoscopic restorative proctocolectomy: an alternative to the conventional approach? *Diseases of the colon and rectum* 45(2): 207-210; discussion 210-201.

Larson, D. W., Dozois, E. J., Piotrowicz, K., Cima, R. R., Wolff, B. G., & Young-Fadok, T. M. (2005). Laparoscopic-assisted vs. open ileal pouch-anal anastomosis: functional outcome in a case-matched series. *Dis Colon Rectum* 48(10): 1845-1850.

Lichtiger, S., Present, D. H., Kornbluth, A., Gelernt, I., Bauer, J., Galler, G., Michelassi, F., & Hanauer, S. (1994). Cyclosporine in severe ulcerative colitis refractory to steroid therapy. *New Engl J Med* 330(26): 1841-1845.

Maggiori, L., Bretagnol, F., Alves, A., & Panis, Y. (2010). Laparoscopic subtotal colectomy for acute or severe colitis with double-end ileo-sigmoidostomy in right iliac fossa. *Surg Laparosc Endosc Percutan Tech* 20(1): 27-29.

Marceau, C., Alves, A., Ouaissi, M., Bouhnik, Y., Valleur, P., & Panis, Y. (2007). Laparoscopic subtotal colectomy for acute or severe colitis complicating inflammatory bowel disease: a case-matched study in 88 patients. *Surgery* 141(5): 640-644.

Marcello, P. W., Milsom, J. W., Wong, S. K., Hammerhofer, K. A., Goormastic, M., Church, J. M., & Fazio, V. W. (2000). Laparoscopic restorative proctocolectomy: case-matched comparative study with open restorative proctocolectomy. *Dis Colon Rectum* 43(5): 604-608.

Nakajima, K., Lee, S. W., Cocilovo, C., Foglia, C., Kim, K., Sonoda, T., & Milsom, J. W. (2004). Hand-assisted laparoscopic colorectal surgery using GelPort. *Surg Endosc* 18(1): 102-105.

Peters, W. R. (1992). Laparoscopic total proctocolectomy with creation of ileostomy for ulcerative colitis: report of two cases. *Journal of laparoendoscopic surgery* 2(3): 175-178.

Rivadeneira, D. E., Marcello, P. W., Roberts, P. L., Rusin, L. C., Murray, J. J., Coller, J. A., & Schoetz, D. J., Jr. (2004). Benefits of hand-assisted laparoscopic restorative proctocolectomy: a comparative study. *Dis Colon Rectum* 47(8): 1371-1376.

Sawada, K., Ohnishi, K., Fukui, S., Yamada, K., Yamamura, M., Amano, K., Wada, M., Tanida, N., & Satomi, M. (1995). Leukocytapheresis therapy, performed with leukocyte removal filter, for inflammatory bowel disease. *J Gastroenterol* 30(3): 322-329.

Seshadri, P. A., Poulin, E. C., Schlachta, C. M., Cadeddu, M. O., & Mamazza, J. (2001). Does a laparoscopic approach to total abdominal colectomy and proctocolectomy offer advantages? *Surg Endosc* 15(8): 837-842.

Sood, A., Midha, V., Sood, N., & Awasthi, G. (2002). A prospective, open-label trial assessing dexamethasone pulse therapy in moderate to severe ulcerative colitis." *J Clin Gastroenterol* 35(4): 328-331.

Telem, D. A., Vine, A. J., Swain, G., Divino, C. M., Salky, B. Greenstein, A. J., Harris, M., & Katz, L. B. (2010). Laparoscopic subtotal colectomy for medically refractory ulcerative colitis: the time has come. *Surg Endosc* 24(7): 1616-1620.

Truelove, S. & Witts L. (1955). Cortisone in ulcerative colitis; final report on a therapeutic trial. *British medical journal* 2(4947): 1041-1048.

Truelove, S. C., & Jewell D. P. (1974). Intensive intravenous regimen for severe attacks of ulcerative colitis. *Lancet* 1(7866): 1067-1070.

Watanabe, K., Funayama, Y., Fukushima, K., Shibata, C., Takahashi, K., & Sasaki, I. (2009). Hand-assisted laparoscopic vs. open subtotal colectomy for severe ulcerative colitis. *Dis Colon Rectum* 52(4): 640-645.

Wexner, S. D., Johansen, O. B., Nogueras, J. J., & Jagelman, D. G. (1992). Laparoscopic total abdominal colectomy. A prospective trial. *Dis Colon Rectum* 35(7): 651-655.

3

Drug Therapy in Ulcerative Colitis

Xue-Gang Guo, Xiang-Ping Wang and Chang-Tai Xu
Xijing Hospital of Digestive Disease,
Editorial Office of Chinese Journal of Neuroanatomy,
Fourth Military Medical University, Xi'an, Shaanxi Province
China

1. Introduction

The two primary types of inflammatory bowel disease (IBD) are ulcerative colitis (CU) and Crohn's disease (CD). These two diseases have many similarities and sometimes are difficult to distinguish from each other. However, there are several differences. UC is an inflammatory destructive disease of the large intestine characterized by motility and secretion disorders. Inflammation usually occurs in the rectum and lower part of the colon, but it may affect the entire colon. UC rarely affects the small intestine except for the end section, called the terminal ileum. UC may also be called colitis or proctitis. Inflammation makes the colon empty frequently, causing diarrhea. Ulcers formed in places where the inflammation has killed the cells of colon, bleeding ulcers and pus discharge. UC is an IBD that causes inflammation in the small intestine and colon. UC can be difficult to diagnose because its symptoms are similar to other intestinal disorders and another type of IBD called CD. CD differs from UC because it causes deeper inflammation within the intestinal wall. Also, CD usually occurs in the small intestine, although it can also occur in the mouth, esophagus, stomach, duodenum, large intestine, appendix, and anus. UC may occur in people of any age, but most often it starts between ages of 15 and 30, or less frequently between ages of 50 and 70. Children and adolescents sometimes develop the disease. UC affects men and women equally and appears to run in some families. Clinical and epidemiological data do not support a simple Mendelian model of inheritance for IBD. In its place CD and UC are considered to be complex polygenic diseases. UC is a chronic disease in which the large intestine becomes inflamed and ulcerated (pitted or eroded), leading to flare-ups (bouts or attacks) of bloody diarrhea, abdominal cramps, and fever. The long-term risk of colon cancer is increased [1-4].

The etiology is unknown for ulcerative colitis (UC). The consensus is so far that it is a response to environmental triggers (infection, drugs, or other agents) in genetically susceptible individuals. The genetic component is not as strong in UC as it is in CD. However, 10%-20% of patients with UC have at least one family member with IBD [1,2]. There are marked differences between ethnic groups with some (such as Ashkenazi Jews) having a particularly high incidence. Non-steroidal anti-inflammatory drugs may cause an episode of acute active disease in some patients with IBD. UC primarily affects young adults, but it can occur at any age from five to eighty years and women tend to be more commonly affected than men. It is a worldwide disorder with high-incidence areas that include United Kingdom, the United States, northern Europe and Australia. Low-incidence

areas include Asia, Japan, and South America. The causes of UC remain unknown. The major theories include infection, allergy to food component, genetics, environmental factors, and immune response to bacteria or other antigens [1]. Typical symptoms during flare-ups include abdominal cramps, an urge to move the bowels, and diarrhea (typically bloody). The diagnosis is based on an examination of the sigmoid colon using a flexible viewing tube (sigmoidoscopy) or an examination of the large intestine using a flexible viewing tube (colonoscopy). People who have had UC for a long time may develop colon cancer. Treatment is aimed at controlling the inflammation, reducing symptoms, and replacing any lost fluids and nutrients. UC may start at any age but usually begins between the ages of 15 and 30. A small group of people have their first attack between the ages of 50 and 70. UC usually does not affect the full thickness of the wall of the large intestine and hardly ever affects the small intestine. The disease usually begins in the rectum or the rectum and the sigmoid colon (the lower end of the large intestine) but may eventually spread along part or all of the large intestine. UC, which is confined to the rectum, is a very common and relatively benign form of UC. In some people, most of the large intestine is affected early on. Ulcerative colitis (UC) affects about one in 1000 people in the Western world. Peak incidence is between the ages of 10 and 40 years. UC may affect people of any age and 15% of people are over the age of 60 at diagnosis [1-4]. The incidence of UC in North America is 10-12 cases per 100,000, with a peak incidence of UC occurring between the ages of 15 and 25. There is thought to be a bimodal distribution in age of onset, with a second peak in incidence occurring in the 6th decade of life. The disease affects females more than males with highest incidences in the United States, Canada, the United Kingdom, and Scandinavia. Higher incidences are seen in northern locations compared to southern locations in Europe and the United States.
Epidemiologic data support genetic contribution to the pathogenesis of IBD. Recently, numerous new genes have been identified to be involved in the genetic susceptibility to IBD [5]: TNF-308A, CARD15 (NOD2), MIF-173 gene, N-acetyltransferase 2 (NAT2), NKG2D (natural killer cell 2D), STAT6 (signal transducer and activator of transcription 6), CTLA-4 (cytotoxic T lymphocyte antigen-4), MICA-MICB (major histocompatibility complex A and B), HLA-DRB1 gene, HLA class-II gene, IL-18 gene (interleukin-18 gene), IL-4 gene, MICA-A5, CD14 gene, TLR4 gene, Fas-670 gene, p53 gene and NF-kappaB. The characterization of these novel genes is potential to identify therapeutic agents and clinical assessment of phenotype and prognosis in patients with IBD (UC and CD). The diagnosis of UC is made from the patient's medical history, a stool examination, sigmoidoscopy findings, and biopsy of specimens from the rectum or colon.

2. Drug treatment

The goals of treatment of UC are to induce and maintain remission of symptoms and inflammation of the inner lining of colon [2, 4, 6, 7]. Treatment options are determined according to the extent of the inflammation and the severity of the disease. Some people have long periods of remission, which can last for years. Unfortunately, the disease usually recurs periodically during an individual's lifetime. Predicting when a flare-up may occur is not possible, but early recognition of symptoms results in a better response to treatment. Patients with this disease are divided into three groups based on the site of involvement, which is important for treatment and prognosis. (1) Proctitis (involving the rectum, the last part of the colon near the anus); (2) Left-sided colitis (from the rectum to the splenic flexure – the area below the ribs on the left side); (3) Pancolitis (involvement more extensive than the above two). Therapy for UC is aimed at quieting inflammation or relieving symptoms. It can usually control symptoms, but surgery may be required when conservative therapy fails or if signs of colon cancer develop.

Both medications and surgery have been used to treat UC. However, surgery is reserved for those with severe inflammation and life-threatening complications. There is no medication so far that can cure UC. Patients with UC will typically experience periods of relapse (worsening of inflammation) followed by periods of remission lasting for months to years. During relapses, symptoms of abdominal pain, diarrhea, and rectal bleeding can worsen patients' quality of life. During remissions, these symptoms subside. Remissions usually occur because of treatment with medications or surgery, but occasionally they occur spontaneously. Since UC cannot be cured by medications, the goals of treatment with medications are to induce remissions, maintain remissions, minimize side effects of drugs, and improve the quality of life. The treatment of UC with medications is similar, though not always identical, to the treatment of CD. Medications treating UC include anti-inflammatory agents such as 5-ASA compounds, systemic and topical corticosteroids, and immunomodulators [2, 8-10].

Anti-inflammatory medications that decrease intestinal inflammation are analogous to arthritis medications that decrease joint inflammation (arthritis). The anti-inflammatory medications used in the treatment of UC are topical 5-ASA compounds such as sulfasalazine (Azulfidine), olsalazine (Dipentum), and mesalamine (Pentasa, Asacol, Rowasa enema) that need direct contact with the inflamed tissues in order to be effective. Systemic corticosteroids can decrease the inflammation throughout the body without direct contact with the inflamed tissue. Systemic corticosteroids have predictable side effects in long-term treatment. Immunomodulators are medications that suppress the body's immune system either by reducing the cells that are responsible for immunity, or by interfering with proteins that are important in promoting inflammation. Immunomodulators are increasingly becoming important for patients with severe UC who do not respond adequately to anti-inflammatory agents. Examples of immunomodulators include 6-mercaptopurine (6-MP), azathioprine, methotrexate, and cyclosporine. There are drugs (including selected side effects and comments) that reduce bowel inflammation in Table 1[2, 8-11].

2.1 Anti-inflammatory drugs

Anti-inflammatory drugs are often the first step in the treatment of UC. Sulfasalazine (Azulfidine) can be effective in reducing symptoms of ulcerative colitis, but it has a number of side effects, including nausea, vomiting, heartburn and headache. This medication can not be given if the patients are allergic to sulfa medications. To evaluate the role of multi-matrix system (MMX) mesalamine in the treatment of UC, literature was obtained through searches of MEDLINE (1966-October 2007) and a bibliographic review of published articles. Key terms used in the searches included UC, mesalamine, MMX, SPD476, and Lialda. All English-language articles that were identified through the search were evaluated. The standard treatment for the induction and maintenance of remission in patients with mild-to-moderate UC is aminosalicylate products (mesalamine, sulfasalazine, balasalazide, olsalazine). Current mesalamine formulations are not ideal for long-term treatment due to issues with patient adherence secondary to complex dosing regimens and high pill burden. Clinical studies show that MMX mesalamine achieves clinical and endoscopic remission more frequently compared with placebo or mesalamine enema. Therefore, MMX mesalamine is an option in patients with UC. The cost of MMX mesalamine is comparable to that of oral and rectal formulations of mesalamine [11, 12].

Drugs	Selected Side Effects	Comments
Aminosalicylates		
Sulfasalazine	Common: Nausea, headache, dizziness, fatigue, fever, rash, reversible male infertility. Uncommon: Inflammation of the liver (hepatitis), pancreas (pancreatitis), or lung (pneumonitis); hemolytic anemia.	Abdominal pain, dizziness, and fatigue are related to dose; hepatitis and pancreatitis are unrelated to dose.
Balsalazide Mesalamine Olsalazine	Common: Fever, rash. Uncommon: Pancreatitis, inflammation of the pericardium (pericarditis), pneumonitis For olsalazine: Watery diarrhea.	Most side effects seen with sulfasalazine may occur with any of the other aminosalicylates but much less frequently.
Corticosteroids		
Prednisone	Diabetes mellitus, high blood pressure, cataracts, osteoporosis, thinning of skin, mental problems, acute psychosis, mood swings, infections, acne, excessive body hair (hirsutism), menstrual irregularities, gastritis, peptic ulcer disease.	Diabetes and high blood pressure are more likely to occur in people who have other risk factors.
Budesonide	Diabetes mellitus, high blood pressure, cataracts, osteoporosis (decreased bone density).	Same side effects as prednisone but to a lesser degree.
Immunomodulators		
Azathioprine Mercaptopurine	Anorexia, nausea, vomiting, infection, cancer, allergic reactions, pancreatitis, low white blood cell count, bone marrow suppression, liver dysfunction.	Side effects that are usually dose dependent include bone marrow suppression and liver dysfunction Interval blood monitoring is required.
Cyclosporine	High blood pressure, nausea, vomiting, diarrhea, kidney failure, tremors, infections, seizures, neuropathy, development of lymphomas (cancers of the lymphatic system).	Side effects become more likely with long-term use.
Methotrexate	Nausea, vomiting, abdominal distress, headache, rash, soreness of the mouth, fatigue, scarring of the liver (cirrhosis), low white blood cell count, infections. Causes abortions and birth defects during pregnancy.	Liver toxicity is likely dose dependent Not prescribed for pregnant women.

Drugs	Selected Side Effects	Comments
Infliximab	Infusion reactions, infections, cancer, abdominal pain, liver dysfunction, low white blood cell count.	Infusion reactions are potential immediate side effects that occur during the infusion such as fever, chills, hives, decreased blood pressure, or difficulty breathing. Patients should be screened for tuberculosis before initiating treatment.
Adalimumab	Pain or itching at the injection site, headache, infections, cancer, and hypersensitivity reactions.	Side effect are similar to infliximab except does not cause infusion reactions. Hypersensitive reactions include rash, urticaria, pruritis, and hives.

Table 1. Drugs selected side effects for therapy UC

Antibiotic therapy may induce remission in active CD and UC, although the diverse number of antibiotics tested means the data are difficult to interpret. This systematic review is a
To systematically evaluate the efficacy of antibacterial therapy in ulcerative colitis, Rahimi et al [15] carried out a meta analysis of controlled clinical trials. Within the time period 1966 through September 2006, PUBMED, EMBASE, and SCOPUS were searched for clinical trial studies that investigated the efficacy of antibiotics in ulcerative colitis. These results suggest that adjunctive antibacterial therapy is effective for induction of clinical remission in UC.
Mesalamine is used to treat ulcerative colitis (a condition in which part or all of the lining of the colon [large intestine] is swollen or worn away). Mesalamine delayed-release tablets and controlled-release capsules may be used to treat ulcerative colitis that affects any part of the colon. Mesalamine suppositories and enemas should only be used to treat inflammation of the lower part of the colon. Mesalamine is in a class of medications called anti-inflammatory agents. It works by stopping the body from producing a certain substance that may cause pain or inflammation. Mesalamine (Asacol, Rowasa) and olsalazine (Dipentum) tend to have fewer side effects than sulfasalazine has. The patients with UC take them in tablet form or use them rectally in the form of enemas or suppositories, depending on the area of the colon affected by ulcerative colitis. Mesalamine enemas can relieve signs and symptoms in more than 80 percent of people with ulcerative colitis in the lower left side of their colon and rectum. Olsalazine may cause or worsen existing diarrhea in some people [2-4].
Balsalazide is more effective than mesalazine in induction of remission, but balsalazide has no benefit compared with mesalazine in preventing relapse in the population selected. The number of patients with any adverse events and withdrawals because of severe adverse events is similar for mesalazine and balsalazide [16].
Articles cited were identified *via* a PubMed search, utilizing the words IBD, adherence, compliance, medication and UC. Medication non-adherence is multifactorial involving factors other than dosing frequency. Male gender (OR: 2.06), new patient status (OR: 2.14), work and travel pressures (OR: 4.9) and shorter disease duration (OR: 2.1), among others are

proven predictors of non-adherence in UC. These indicators can identify 'at-risk' patients and allow an individually tailored treatment approach to be introduced that optimizes medication adherence. A collaborative relationship between physician and patient is important. Several strategies for improving adherence have been proven effective including open dialogue that consideration the patient's health beliefs and concerns, providing educational (e.g. verbal/written information, self-management programmes) and behavioural interventions (e.g. calendar blister packs, cues/reminders). Hawthorne *et al* [17] considered that educational and behavioural interventions tailored to individual patients can optimize medication adherence. Additional studies combining educational and behavioural interventions may provide further strategies for improving medication adherence rates in UC. Swaminath *et al* [18] reviews current data to optimize the use of both older and newer drugs in inflammatory bowel disease. For patients with severe UC, steroid dosing has been clarified, and a mega-analysis of steroid outcomes and toxicities has been reported. In regard to mesalamine, recent information has suggested benefit of a higher dose of pH-dependent release mesalamine for patients with moderate UC. Also, a once-daily formulation with multi-matrix system (MMX) technology (Shire Pharmaceuticals, Wayne, PA), has been approved. In regard to cyclosporine, two centers have reported an increased rate of colectomy over a long-duration follow-up of a cyclosporine course given for UC. Additional information regarding thiopurines has been published, including the use of metabolite testing and duration of therapy for these drugs [19, 20].
5-aminosalicylic acids (5-ASAs), a number of oral 5-ASA agents are commercially available, including azo-bond pro-drugs such as sulfasalazine, olsalazine and balsalazide, and delayed- and controlled-release forms of mesalazine [12, 21, 22]. The effectiveness of oral therapy relies on good compliance, which may be adversely affected by frequent daily dosing and a large number of tablets. Furthermore, poor adherence has been shown to be an important barrier to successful management of patients with UC. Recently, new, once-daily formulations of mesalazine including the unique multi-matrix delivery system and mesalazine granules were proven to be efficacious in inducing and maintaining remission in mild-to-moderate UC, with a good safety profile comparable to that of other oral mesalazine formulations. The advantage of low pill burden may contribute to increased long-term compliance and treatment success in clinical practice and might potentially further contribute to a decline in the risk for UC-associated colon cancers. In this systematic review, Lakatos *et al* [19] summarized the available literature on the short- and medium-term efficacy and safety of the new once-daily mesalazine formulations.
5-ASA agents are the first-line therapy for UC. A high-dose, once-daily formulation of 5-ASA known as MMX mesalamine has recently been approved for the treatment of UC. A systematic review of published literature was performed on PubMed using the search terms 'MMX mesalamine' and 'Lialda'. Abstracts presented at US gastroenterology conferences between 2006 and 2007, were also reviewed. MMX mesalamine uses a novel multi-matrix delivery system to achieve a sustained release of 5-ASA throughout the colon. Clinical trials have demonstrated that MMX mesalamine 2.4 g/day or 4.8 g/day is superior to placebo in inducing remission in active mild to moderate UC. The drug is well tolerated with a safety profile comparable to other oral 5-ASAs agents. With a high-dose formulation of 1.2 g 5-ASA per tablet, MMX mesalamine can be administered conveniently at two to four pills once a day. MMX mesalamine is the first and only approved once-daily 5-ASAs treatment option for patients with UC. It is efficacious for the induction of remission in mild to moderate UC and

has a favorable safety profile. With the advantage of low pill burden and easy dosing schedule, it may potentially improve patient compliance and treatment success [20].

The efficacy of 5-ASAs in ulcerative colitis (UC) has been studied previously in meta-analyses. However, several randomized controlled trials (RCTs) have been published recently, and no previous meta-analysis has studied the effect of 5-ASA dosage used. Ford *et al* [23] suggested that 5-ASAs are highly effective for inducing remission and preventing relapse in UC. Evidence suggests that 5-ASA doses of ≥2.0 g/day have greater efficacy, although doses >2.5 g/day do not appear to lead to higher remission rates.

Sulfasalazine (SSZ) does not differ from mesalamine or olsalazine in terms of efficacy and tolerability in UC. Withdrawal from study due to adverse events was significantly lower for balsalazide compared with SSZ. Convincing conclusions on the comparison of effectiveness and safety of balsalazide and SSZ in UC remains to be elucidated by further clinical trials. Considering the lower cost of treatment with SSZ and the equal rate of adverse events with other 5-ASAa, it is not surprising to suggest SSZ as a first-choice treatment for UC and reserve 5-ASAs for when SSZ intolerability occurs [24].

Ulcerative proctitis (UP) is a common presentation of UC. Extensive Medline/Embase literature search was performed to identify relevant articles. Topical medication with rectally administered 5-ASA/corticosteroid suppositories or enemas is an effective treatment for most UP patients. Locally administered 5-ASA is more efficacious than oral compounds. The combination of topical 5-ASA and oral 5-ASA or topical steroids should be considered for escalation of treatment. Maintenance treatment is indicated in all UC cases. 5-ASA suppositories are suggested as first-line maintenance therapy if accepted by patients, although oral 5-ASA as maintenance therapy might prevent proximal extension of the disease. After re-assessment, chronically active patients refractory or intolerant to 5-ASAs and corticosteroids may require immunomodulators or biological therapy [12, 20-23]. Rectal 5-ASA should be considered a first-line therapy for patients with mild to moderately active distal UC. The optimal total daily dose and dose frequency of 5-ASA remain to be determined. Future research should define differences in efficacy among patient subgroups defined by proximal disease margin and disease activity. There is a strong need for consensus standardization of outcome measurements for clinical trials in ulcerative colitis [25]..

Infliximab is effective for treatment of moderate-to-severe UC and is recommended for patients who have had an inadequate response to medical therapy or who are intolerant of or do not desire to take the potential risk of using specific agents including immunomodulators (cyclosporine A, azathioprine, or 6-mercaptopurine), corticosteroids, and, potentially, mesalamine. Future trials are needed to assess the efficacy of infliximab with immunomodulators to see if additional benefit is achieved so that the risk-benefit ratio is positive. Based on the favorable efficacy of infliximab for UC therapy, the ground work has been established for evaluating infliximab and addressing some of the many unanswered questions and also for assessing other anti-TNF agents and streamlining the anti-TNG antibody to improve efficacy, reduce side effects, and ease administration [22]. Infliximab (Remicade) is specifically for adults and children with moderate to severe ulcerative colitis who don't respond to or can't tolerate other treatments. The drug has been linked to an increased risk of infection, especially tuberculosis, and may increase your risk of blood problems and cancer. Before taking infliximab a skin test for tuberculosis and a chest X-ray are necessary if the patients lived or traveled extensively where tuberculosis has been found. Also, because Remicade contains mouse protein, it can cause serious allergic reactions in some people — reactions that may be delayed for days to weeks after starting treatment. Once started, infliximab is often continued as long-term therapy, although its effectiveness may wear off over time.

2.2 Corticosteroids

Corticosteroids can help reduce inflammation, but they have numerous side effects, including a puffy face, excessive facial hair, night sweats, insomnia and hyperactivity. Long-term use of these drugs in children can lead to stunted growth. Also, corticosteroids don't work for everyone who has ulcerative colitis. Doctors generally use corticosteroids only if you have moderate to severe inflammatory bowel disease that doesn't respond to other treatments. Corticosteroids aren't for long-term use and are generally prescribed for a period of three to four months. They may also be used in conjunction with other medications as a means to induce remission. These, too, are only for short-term use [2, 8].

MEDLINE, EMBASE, and the Cochrane central register of controlled trials were searched (through December 2010) by Ford *et al* [26]. Randomized controlled trials (RCTs) recruiting adults with active or quiescent CD comparing standard glucocorticosteroids or budesonide with placebo or each other, or comparing standard glucocorticosteroids with placebo in active UC, were eligible. Dichotomous data were extracted to obtain relative risk (RR) of failure to achieve remission in active disease, and RR of relapse of activity in quiescent disease, with a 95% confidence interval (CI). Adverse events data were extracted where reported. Standard glucocorticosteroids are probably effective in inducing remission in UC, and may be of benefit in CD. Budesonide induces remission in active CD, but is less effective than standard glucocorticosteroids, and is of no benefit in preventing CD relapse.

Recent progress in both basic and clinical research has led us to develop sophisticated and effective medical therapy of UC. Although classical agents such as aminosalicylates, corticosteroids and immunomodulatory drugs have remained as the gold standard for decades, their novel formulations and/or dosage regimens have changed their placements in the medical management of UC. In addition, studies have shown that a number of novel therapeutic agents, designed to target specific mechanisms involved in the inflammatory cascade, have efficacy for the treatment of UC and they will have significant clinical impacts in the near future. A clear understanding of the proven and potential benefits of both the standard and emerging therapies will be required for the optimum individual care of patients with varied clinical presentations [12, 18, 27-29].

2.3 Immune system suppressors

These drugs also reduce inflammation, but they target the immune system rather than inflammation itself. Because immune suppressors can be effective in treating ulcerative colitis, scientists theorize that damage of the digestive tissues is caused by the body's immune response to an invading virus or bacterium or even to patients own tissue. By suppressing this response, inflammation is also reduced. Azathioprine (Imuran) and mercaptopurine (Purinethol) have been used to treat CD and UC for years, but their role in ulcerative colitis is only now being studied. Because azathioprine and mercaptopurine act slowly, they're sometimes initially combined with a corticosteroid, but in time, they seem to produce benefits on their own, with less long-term toxicity. Side effects can include allergic reactions, bone marrow suppression, infections, and inflammation of the liver and pancreas. If a patient is taking either of these medications, he or she'll need to follow up closely with his or her doctor and have your blood checked regularly to look for side effects.

Cyclosporine (Neoral, Sandimmune), a potent drug, is normally reserved for people who don't respond well to other medications or who face surgery because of severe UC.

Published trials evaluating the efficacy of 6-thioguanine anti-metabolites in the treatment of UC have yielded conflicting results. Leung *et al* [30] performed a systematic review and meta-analysis to evaluate the clinical efficacy of 6-thioguanine anti-metabolites for the maintenance of clinical remission after standard induction with corticosteroids. A comprehensive search of online databases was conducted. Only randomized controlled trials with 6-thioguanine antimetabolites within a minimum duration of follow-up of 6 months were selected. Five trials were included in the meta-analysis. Pooled results demonstrated a modest efficacy of azathioprine (AZA) for the treatment of ulcerative colitis. However, the use of AZA for the management of UC is not based on high-quality evidence.

There remains controversy regarding the efficacy of thiopurine analogs (AZA and 6-MP), methotrexate (MTX), and cyclosporine for the treatment of inflammatory bowel disease (IBD). An updated systematic review of the literature to clarify the efficacy of immunosuppressive therapy at inducing remission and preventing relapse in UC and CD was performed. Most evidence relates to AZA/6-MP where there is no statistically significant benefit at inducing remission in active CD and UC. Thiopurine analogs may prevent relapse in quiescent UC and CD. However, there is a paucity of data for immunosuppressive therapy in IBD and more research is needed [31].

Over the last decade, the increasing knowledge on the pathogenic mechanisms underlying intestinal inflammation has led to the development of a number of biological agents, mainly addressed to molecules and/or pathways demonstrated to have a pathogenic role in UC. In UC, clinical course and therapeutic decisions mainly depend on disease activity and extent. While therapeutic approach to mild-to-moderate UC by using aminosalicylates and corticosteroids has been well established, treatment of severe UC is far from being satisfactory. A severe attack of UC remains a challenge to be managed jointly by gastroenterology, surgery, and intensive care units. However, the recent introduction of biological therapies has led to promising changes in the management of UC patients. Aim of this paper is to review the recent advances and future perspectives for the use of biological agents in UC [32, 33]. Side effects of cyclosporine include high blood pressure, renal function impairment, and tingling sensations in the extremities. More serous side effects include anaphylactic shock and seizures.

Mucosal macrophages play an important role in the mucosal immune system, and an increase in the number of newly recruited monocytes and activated macrophages has been noted in the inflamed gut of patients with IBD. Activated macrophages are thought to be major contributors to the production of inflammatory cytokines in the gut, and imbalance of cytokines is contributing to the pathogenesis of IBD. The intestinal inflammation in IBD is controlled by a complex interplay of innate and adaptive immune mechanisms. Cytokines play a key role in IBD that determine T cell differentiation of Th1, Th2, T regulatory and newly described Th17 cells. Cytokines levels in time and space orchestrate the development, recurrence and exacerbation of the inflammatory process in IBD [34-36].

Progress has occurred in all major areas relevant to IBD pathogenesis, which include the external environment, genetics, microbial factors, and the immune system. This review presents an update on the specific major advances that have occurred in each of these four areas, briefly discusses the therapeutic implications of the observed progress, and points out the additional work that needs to be accomplished in the next few years to reach a full understanding of IBD etiopathogenesis [35,36].

VSL#3 (VSL#3) is a high-concentration probiotic preparation of eight live freeze-dried bacterial species that are normal components of the human gastrointestinal microflora, including four strains of lactobacilli (*Lactobacillus casei, L. plantarum, L. acidophilus,* and *L. delbrueckii* subsp. *bulgaricus*), three strains of bifidobacteria, and *Streptococcus salivarius* subsp. thermophilus. Data from noncomparative trials suggest that VSL#3 has clinical potential in the treatment of active mild to moderate ulcerative colitis and as maintenance therapy for patients with ulcerative colitis in remission. In addition, a randomized, open-labelled, multicenter trial showed that VSL#3 in combination with low-dose balsalazide (a prodrug of mesalazine [mesalamine; 5-ASA]) was more effective than standard doses of basalazide or mesalazine monotherapy in the treatment of acute mild to moderate ulcerative colitis. Randomized, double-blind, placebo-controlled studies have shown that VSL#3 is effective in preventing the onset of acute pouchitis in patients with newly formed surgical pouches, and in maintaining remission following antibacterial treatment of acute pouchitis in patients with a history of refractory or recurrent pouchitis. Treatment guidelines from the US and the UK include VSL#3 as a therapeutic option for the prevention of pouchitis relapse in patients with chronic pouchitis. In general, VSL#3 was well tolerated in clinical trials. Large, well designed, controlled confirmatory clinical trials will further determine the place of VSL#3 in the treatment of UC [18].

2.4 Nicotine

The skin patches seem to provide short-term relief from flare-ups of UC for some people, especially people who formerly smoked. How nicotine patches work isn't exactly clear, and the evidence that they provide relief is contested among researchers.

UC is characterized by impairment of the epithelial barrier and the formation of ulcer-type lesions, which result in local leaks and generalized alterations of mucosal tight junctions. Ultimately, this results in increased basal permeability. Although disruption of the epithelial barrier in the gut is a hallmark of inflammatory bowel disease and intestinal infections, it remains unclear whether barrier breakdown is an initiating event of UC or rather a consequence of an underlying inflammation, evidenced by increased production of proinflammatory cytokines. UC is less common in smokers, suggesting that the nicotine in cigarettes may ameliorate disease severity. The mechanism behind this therapeutic effect is still not fully understood, and indeed it remains unclear if nicotine is the true protective agent in cigarettes. Nicotine is metabolized in the body into a variety of metabolites and can also be degraded to form various breakdown products. Possibly, these metabolites or degradation products may be the true protective or curative agents. A greater understanding of the pharmacodynamics and kinetics of nicotine in relation to the immune system and enhanced knowledge of gut permeability defects in UC are required to establish the exact protective nature of nicotine and its metabolites in UC. This review suggests possible hypotheses for the protective mechanism of nicotine in UC, highlight the relationship between gut permeability and inflammation, and indicates where in the pathogenesis of the disease nicotine may mediate its effect [1-3, 12-14].

UC is predominantly a disease of non-smokers, and nicotine may be the agent responsible for this association. Transdermal nicotine has been shown to improve disease activity and sigmoidoscopic appearance in the active disease, but in one study it had no effect on maintenance of remission. Since side-effects with nicotine patches occur in up to two thirds of patients, attempts to reduce systemic levels and improve drug tolerance have been developed with colonic delivery systems of nicotine. Preliminary observations with nicotine enemas in UC have shown clinical benefit, but controlled trials are needed. Mechanisms responsible for the association of smoking with colitis and for the therapeutic effect of nicotine remain an enigma; possibilities include: modulation of the immune response, alterations of colonic mucus and eicosanoid production, changes in rectal blood flow, decreased intestinal permeability and the release of endogenous glucocorticoids [19-22].

Smoking has been associated with a decreased frequency of UC. Currently, the role of nicotine for the treatment of UC is not established. Several studies have evaluated nicotine gum and transdermal patches as supplemental therapy for stable UC, but nicotine has not been compared with other treatment modalities. Nicotine dosages in the studies have varied from 5 to 30 mg/d without apparent dose-related therapeutic effects, and many patients have found relief from placebo treatment. Patients often do not tolerate nicotine therapy's adverse effects, such as nausea, light-headedness, and headache. Due to the cyclic disease course of UC and the potential addictiveness of nicotine, further large studies are warranted to assess the benefits of nicotine therapy for UC [29].

There are significant proportions of patients with UC who experience adverse effects with current therapies. Consequently, new alternatives for the treatment of UC are constantly being sought. Probiotics are live microbial feed supplements that may beneficially affect the host by improving intestinal microbial balance, enhancing gut barrier function and improving local immune response. Mallon *et al* [12] assessed the efficacy of probiotics compared with placebo or standard medical treatment (5-aminosalicylates, sulfasalazine or corticosteroids) for the induction of remission in active ulcerative colitis. A comprehensive search for relevant randomised controlled trials (RCT's) was carried out using MEDLINE (1966-January 2006), EMBASE (January 1985- 2006) and CENTRAL. The Cochrane IBD/FBD Review Group Specialised Trials Registrar was also searched. The Australasian Medical Index, Chinese Biomedical Literature Database, Latin American Caribbean Health Sciences Literature (LILACS), and the Japan Information Centre of Science and Technology File on Science, Technology and Medicine (JICST-E) were also used to identify abstracts. Conference proceedings from the Falk Symposium, Digestive Disease Week (DDW) and the United European Digestive Disease week were hand-searched. Authors of relevant studies and drug companies were contacted regarding ongoing or unpublished trials that may be relevant to the review. However, there is limited evidence that probiotics added to standard therapy may provide modest benefits in terms of reduction of disease activity in patients with mild to moderately severe UC. Whether probiotics are as effective in patients with severe and more extensive disease and whether they can be used as an alternative to existing therapies is unknown [12].

2.5 Heparin

Heparin is a naturally-occurring anticoagulant produced by basophils and mast cells. Heparin acts as an anticoagulant, preventing the formation of clots and extension of existing clots within the blood. While heparin does not break down clots that have already formed (unlike tissue plasminogen activator), it allows the body's natural clot lysis mechanisms to work normally to break down clots that have formed.

An increased risk of thrombosis in UC coupled with an observation that UC patients being treated with anticoagulant therapy for thrombotic events had an improvement in their bowel symptoms led to trials examining the use of unfractionated heparin (UFH) and low molecular weight heparins (LMWH) in patients with active UC. There is evidence to suggest that LMWH may be effective for the treatment of active UC. When administered by extended colon-release tablets, LMWH was more effective than placebo for treating outpatients with mild to moderate disease. This benefit needs to be confirmed by further randomized controlled studies. The same benefits were not seen when LMWH was administered subcutaneously at lower doses. There is no evidence to support the use of UFH for the treatment of active UC. A further trial of UFH in patients with mild disease may also be justified. Any benefit found would need to be weighed against a possible increased risk of rectal bleeding in patients with active UC [37].

2.6 Interferons

Interferons (IFNs) are cytokines which possess immunoregulatory properties and have been used to successfully treat a number of chronic inflammatory disorders. It has been postulated that Type I IFNs may be able to re-establish the Th1/Th2 balance in Th2 predominant diseases like ulcerative colitis.

Seow *et al* [38] reported that four studies were eligible for inclusion. Three studies compared type I IFNs to placebo and a single study compared IFNs to prednisolone enemas in patients with left-sided colitis. Meta-analysis was based on the three IFN-placebo studies. There was no significant benefit of type I IFNs over placebo for inducing remission in ulcerative colitis (RR 1.24; 95% CI 0.81 to 1.90). There were no statistically significant differences in any of the secondary outcome variables. Conclusions were suggested by Seow *et al* [38] that the existing literature does not support the efficacy of type I IFNs for induction of remission in patients with UC. Given concerns regarding the tolerability of IFN therapy, we suggest that the results of two ongoing trials are evaluated for efficacy and safety prior to development or commencement of further randomised controlled trials of type I IFNs in UC.

3. Treatment of traditional Chinese medicine

Traditional Chinese medicine (TCM) believes that the major pathologies of UC include spleen and stomach dysfunctions, intestinal turbid accumulations, and blood and qi disturbances. Therefore, TCM treatment strategies are to restore organ functioning, eliminate turbid accumulations and harmonize the flows of qi and blood. In clinical applications, if individuals have obvious pus, mucus or bloody loose bowels, physicians will focus on clearing pathogens like damp-heat or damp-cold, so as to improve the bowel environment. Afterwards, notifying methods are employed to overcome the internal weakness and promote a longer remission period [2, 39-42].

Chinese medicine is getting more and more popular nowadays in the whole world for improving health condition of human beings as well as preventing and healing diseases. Chinese medicine is a multi-component system with components mostly unknown, and only a few compounds are responsible for the pharmaceutical and/or toxic effects. The large numbers of other components in the Chinese medicine make the screening and analysis of the bioactive components extremely difficult. So, separation and analysis of the desired chemical components in Chinese medicine are very important subjects for modernization research of Chinese medicine. Thus, many novel separation techniques with significant advantages over conventional methods were introduced and applied for separation and analysis of the chemical constituents in Chinese medicine. This review presents just a brief outline of the applications of different separation methods for the isolation and analysis of Chinese medicine constituents [2, 7]. Chinese medicine was widely used in the treatment of

UC. Treatment of chronic UC by traditional Chinese and Western medicine is safe and effective in maintaining remission [39, 40].

Stimulation of acupuncture not only enhances the immune modulation effect, but also mobilizes the innate healing power inside the body. For the localized problems like inflammation, ulcers, muscular spasms and sluggish flow, acupuncture and moxibustion are particularly effective and thus facilitate structural recovery [41, 42]. Major points are navel's four-point (one-thumb-width apart from the navel, located in three, six, nine & twelve o'clock), *tian-shu, guan-yuan* & *qi-hai;* Assist points are *da-chang-shu, zhang-qiang, pi-shu, wei-shu, zu-san-li* & *san-yin-jiao.* When applying, firstly the four-point needle should be punctured in 0.3-0.5 cm deep 30-second for about rotations, with stimulation of the four locations in a clockwise sequence, without needle retention. Then one more major point and 2 to 3 assist points should be selected for stimulation, with the needles retaining on the locations for 15-20 minutes, and the moxa cones can be attached for heating during this time. Procedure is performed once daily or every two days with ten times is one course [2, 42].

Moxibustion can also be used to boost the weakened systems, particularly for individuals with chronic symptoms. Below are suggested protocols. The major points are *zhong-wan, tian-shu, guan-yuan* & *shang-ju-xu, and the* assist points are *pi-shu, shen-shu, da-chang-shu, zu-san-li, tai-xi, tai-chong, san-yin-jiao* & *zhong-iv-shu*. Each time, 1-2 major points should be selected with heat for 30-40 minutes, while 2-3 assist points should be punctured with heat for 15-20 minutes. This procedure is performed once daily or every two days, with 15-20 times in one course.

Acupuncture-type treatments are among the most popular options. Several studies have reported that moxibustion is effective in ulcerative colitis (UC). The objective of this review was to assess the clinical evidence for or against moxibustion as a treatment for UC. Lee *et al* [43] searched the literature using 18 databases from their inception to February 10, 2010, without language restrictions. Randomized clinical trials (RCTs) were included, in which human patients with UC were treated with moxibustion. Studies were included if they were placebo-controlled or controlled against a drug therapy or no treatment group. The methodological quality of all RCTs was assessed using the Cochrane risk of bias. In total, five RCTs were included. All were of low methodological quality. They compared the effects of moxibustion with conventional drug therapy. Three tested moxibustion against sulfasalazine and two against sulfasalazine plus other drugs. A meta-analysis of five RCTs showed favorable effects of moxibustion on the response rate compared to conventional drug therapy ($n = 407$; risk ratio = 1.24, 95% CI = 1.11 to 1.38; $P < 0.0001$; heterogeneity: $I2 = 16\%$). The results showed that current evidence is insufficient to show that moxibustion is an effective treatment of UC. Most of included trials had high risk of bias. More rigorous studies seem warranted.

In addition to controlling inflammation, some medications may help relieve the signs and symptoms. Depending on the severity of UC, the patients are recommended one or more of the following [2, 8, 18-21].

Antidiarrheals: A fiber supplement such as psyllium powder (Metamucil) or methylcellulose (Citrucel) can help relieve signs and symptoms of mild to moderate diarrhea by adding bulk to the stool. For more severe diarrhea, loperamide (Imodium) may be effective. Use anti-diarrheal medications with great caution, however, because they increase the risk of toxic megacolon.

Laxatives: In some cases, swelling may cause the intestines to narrow, leading to constipation.

Pain relievers: For mild pain, the patients recommend acetaminophen (Tylenol, others). Nonsteroidal anti-inflammatory drugs (NSAIDs) should not be applied such as aspirin, ibuprofen (Advil, Motrin, others) or naproxen (Aleve). These are likely to make patient's symptoms worse.

Iron supplements: If patients have chronic intestinal bleeding, they may develop iron deficiency anemia. Taking iron supplements may help restore patient's iron levels to normal and reduce this type of anemia once the bleeding has stopped or diminished.

Parenteral hyperalimentation: For severe UC patients, it is one kind of security, the effective feasible method.

4. Surgery

Surgery is required in the vast majority of patients with CD and in approximately one-third of patients with UC. Similar to medical treatments for IBD, significant advances have occurred in surgery. Advances in CD include an emphasis upon conservatism as exemplified by more limited resections, strictureplasties, and laparoscopic resections. The use of probiotics in selected patients has improved the outcome in patients with pouchitis following restorative proctocolectomy for UC. It is anticipated that ongoing discoveries in the molecular basis of IBD will in turn identify those patients who will best respond to surgery [44]. Emergency surgery may be necessary for acute life-threatening attacks with massive bleeding, perforations, toxic megacolon, or blood clotting. Since the introduction of laparoscopy into colorectal surgery in the early 1990s, almost every procedure was attempted laparoscopically. Consequently, many very experienced surgical groups conducted numerous trials in an attempt to determine whether laparoscopy in IBD is indeed beneficial or not. The focus of this review is minimally invasive procedures in patients with UC [45].

5. Summary

Ulcerative colitis (UC) and Crohn's disease (CD) are two primary types of inflammatory bowel disease (IBD). UC is an inflammatory destructive disease of the large intestine occurred usually in the rectum and lower part of the colon as well as the entire colon. Drug therapy is a main choice for UC treatment and medical management should be as a comprehensive one. Several types of medications are used to control the inflammation or reduce symptoms caused by ulcerative colitis. The treatment of UC depends on its severity, location and the presence of complications, so drug therapies must be custom-designed for each patient. Findings which medications best alleviate the symptoms may take time. The goal of medical treatment is to reduce the inflammation that triggers the signs and symptoms [2-4]. In the best cases, this may lead not only to symptom relief but also to long-term remission. Azulfidine, Asacol, Pentasa, Dipentum, and Rowasa all contain 5-ASA, which is the topical anti-inflammatory ingredient. In UC patients with moderate to severe disease and in patients who failed to respond to 5-ASA compounds, systemic corticosteroids should be used. To minimize side effects, corticosteroids should be gradually reduced as soon as the disease remission is achieved [13-15]. Surgery or immunomodulator is considered for patients with corticosteroid-dependent or unresponsive to corticosteroid treatment. Immunomodulators used for treating severe UC include azathioprine/6-MP, methotrexate, and cyclosporine [46-50]. Integrated traditional Chinese and Western medicine is safe and effective in maintaining remission in patients with UC.

The goal of drug therapy is to induce and maintain remission, and to improve the quality of life for people with ulcerative colitis. Several types of drugs are available. Drug treatment ulcerative colitis includes the following three categories: aminosalicylates, corticosteroids and immunomodulators. Other drugs may be given to relax the patient or to relieve pain, diarrhea, or infection.

5.1 Aminosalicylates

These drugs that contain 5-aminosalicyclic acid (5-ASA) help control inflammation. Sulfasalazine is a combination of sulfapyridine and 5-ASA. The sulfapyridine component carries the anti-inflammatory 5-ASA to the intestine. However, sulfapyridine may lead to side effects such as nausea, vomiting, heartburn, diarrhea, and headache. Other 5-ASA agents, such as olsalazine, mesalamine, and balsalazide, have a different carrier, fewer side effects, and may be used by people who cannot take sulfasalazine. 5-ASAs are given orally, through an enema, or in a suppository, depending on the location of the inflammation in the colon. Most people with mild or moderate ulcerative colitis are treated with this group of drugs first. This class of drugs is also used in cases of relapse.

5.2 Corticosteroids

Corticosteroids such as prednisone, methylprednisone, and hydrocortisone also reduce inflammation. They may be used by patients who have moderate to severe UC or who do not respond to 5-ASA drugs. Corticosteroids, also known as steroids, can be given orally, intravenously, through an enema, or in a suppository, depending on the location of the inflammation. The drugs can cause side effects such as weight gain, acne, facial hair, hypertension, diabetes, mood swings, bone mass loss, and an increased risk of infection. For this reason, they are not recommended for long-term use, although they are considered very effective when prescribed for short-term use.

5.3 Immunomodulators

These drugs such as azathioprine and 6-mercapto-purine (6-MP) reduce inflammation by affecting the immune system. Azathioprine and 6-MP are used for patients who have not responded to 5-ASAs or corticosteroids or who are dependent on corticosteroids. Immunomodulators are administered orally, however, patients are slow-acting and it may take up to 6 months before the full benefit. Patients taking these drugs are monitored for complications including pancreatitis, hepatitis, a reduced white blood cell count, and an increased risk of infection. Cyclosporine A may be used with 6-MP or azathioprine to treat active, severe UC in patients who do not respond to intravenous corticosteroids.

6. References

[1] Kozuch PL, Hanauer SB.Treatment of inflammatory bowel disease: a review of medical therapy. World J Gastroenterol. 2008;14(3):354-77. PMID: 18200659

[2] Xu CT, Meng SY, Pan BR. Drug therapy for ulcerative colitis.World J Gastroenterol. 2004;10(16): 2311-7. PMID: 15285010

[3] Karban A, Eliakim R. Effect of smoking on inflammatory bowel disease: Is it disease or organ specific? World J Gastroenterol. 2007;13(15):2150-2. PMID: 17465492

[4] McGilligan VE, Wallace JM, Heavey PM, Ridley DL, Rowland IR.Hypothesis about mechanisms through which nicotine might exert its effect on the interdependence of inflammation and gut barrier function in ulcerative colitis.Inflamm Bowel Dis. 2007;13(1):108-15. PMID: 17206646

[5] Yun J, Xu CT, Pan BR. Epidemiology and gene markers of ulcerative colitis in the Chinese. World J Gastroenterol. 2009;15(7):788-803. PubMed PMID:19230040; PubMed Central PMCID: PMC2653379

[6] Jiang XL, Cui HF. An analysis of 10218 ulcerative colitis cases in China.World J Gastroenterol. 2002;8(1):158-61.PMID: 11833094

[7] Liu S, Yi LZ, Liang YZ.Traditional Chinese medicine and separation science. J Sep Sci. 2008;31(11): 2113-37. PMID: 18615809

[8] Xu CT, Pan BR.Current medical therapy for ulcerative colitis.World J Gastroenterol. 1999;5(1):64-72. PMID: 11819390

[9] Odes S. How expensive is inflammatory bowel disease? A critical analysis.World J Gastroenterol. 2008; 14(43):6641-7.PMID: 19034966

[10] Jess T. Prognosis of inflammatory bowel disease across time and countries. An epidemiological study of population-based patient cohorts.Dan Med Bull. 2008;55(2):103-20.PMID: 19017498

[11] Kale-Pradhan PB, Pradhan RS, Wilhelm SM.Multi-matrix system mesalamine: to use or not to use. Ann Pharmacother. 2008;42(2):265-9. PMID: 18182473

[12] Mallon P, McKay D, Kirk S, Gardiner K. Probiotics for induction of remission in ulcerative colitis. Cochrane Database Syst Rev. 2007;(4):CD005573. PMID: 17943867

[13] Khan KJ, Ullman TA, Ford AC, Abreu MT, Abadir A, Marshall JK, Talley NJ, Moayyedi P. Antibiotic therapy in inflammatory bowel disease: a systematic review and meta-analysis. Am J Gastroenterol. 2011;106(4):661-73. PubMed PMID: 21407187

[14] Gionchetti P, Rizzello F, Lammers KM, Morselli C, Tambasco R, Campieri M. Antimicrobials in the management of inflammatory bowel disease. Digestion. 2006;73(Suppl 1):77-85. PubMed PMID: 16498255

[15] Rahimi R, Nikfar S, Rezaie A, Abdollahi M. A meta-analysis of antibiotic therapy for active ulcerative colitis. Dig Dis Sci. 2007;52(11):2920-5. PubMed PMID: 17415632

[16] Rahimi R, Nikfar S, Rezaie A, Abdollahi M. Comparison of mesalazine and balsalazide in induction and maintenance of remission in patients with ulcerative colitis: a meta-analysis. Dig Dis Sci. 2009;54(4):712-21. PubMed PMID: 18683049

[17] Hawthorne AB, Rubin G, Ghosh S.Review article: medication non-adherence in ulcerative colitis--strategies to improve adherence with mesalazine and other maintenance therapies. Aliment Pharmacol Ther. 2008;27(12):1157-66. PMID: 18384664

[18] Swaminath A, Kornbluth A. Optimizing drug therapy in inflammatory bowel disease. Curr Gastroenterol Rep. 2007;9(6):513-20. PMID: 18377805

[19] Lakatos PL, Lakatos L. Effectiveness of new, once-daily 5-aminosalicylic acid in the treatment of ulcerative colitis]. Orv Hetil. 2009;150(9):397-404. PubMed PMID: 19228568

[20] Lakatos PL, Lakatos L.Ulcerative proctitis: a review of pharmacotherapy and management.Expert Opin Pharmacother. 2008 Apr;9(5):741-9. PMID: 18345952

[21] Jiang XL, Cui HF. Different therapy for different types of ulcerative colitis in China.World J Gastroenterol. 2004;10(10):1513-20.PMID: 15133864

[22] Aberra FN, Lichtenstein GR.Infliximab in ulcerative colitis.Gastroenterol Clin North Am. 2006;35(4): 821-36. PMID: 17129815
[23] Ford AC, Achkar JP, Khan KJ, Kane SV, Talley NJ, Marshall JK, Moayyedi P. Efficacy of 5-aminosalicylates in ulcerative colitis: systematic review and meta-analysis. Am J Gastroenterol. 2011;106(4):601-16. PubMed PMID: 21407188
[24] Nikfar S, Rahimi R, Rezaie A, Abdollahi M. A meta-analysis of the efficacy of sulfasalazine in comparison with 5-aminosalicylates in the induction of improvement and maintenance of remission in patients with ulcerative colitis. Dig Dis Sci. 2009;54(6):1157-70. PubMed PMID: 18770034
[25] Marshall JK, Thabane M, Steinhart AH, Newman JR, Anand A, Irvine EJ. Rectal 5-aminosalicylic acid for induction of remission in ulcerative colitis. Cochrane Database Syst Rev. 2010;(1):CD004115. PubMed PMID: 20091560
[26] Ford AC, Bernstein CN, Khan KJ, Abreu MT, Marshall JK, Talley NJ, Moayyedi P. Glucocorticosteroid therapy in inflammatory bowel disease: systematic review and meta-analysis. Am J Gastroenterol. 2011;106(4):590-9; quiz 600. PubMed PMID: 21407179
[27] Chapman TM, Plosker GL, Figgitt DP.Spotlight on VSL#3 probiotic mixture in chronic inflammatory bowel diseases. Bio Drugs. 2007;21(1):61-3. PMID: 17263590
[28] Nakamura T, Nagahori M, Kanai T, Watanabe M.Current pharmacologic therapies and emerging alternatives in the treatment of ulcerative colitis.Digestion. 2008;77(Suppl 1):36-41. PMID: 18204260
[29] Cui HH, Chen CL, Wang JD, Yang YJ, Sun Y, Wang YD, Lai ZS.[The effects of bifidobacterium on the intestinal mucosa of the patients with ulcerative colitis.Zhonghua Nei Ke Za Zhi. 2003;42(8):554-7.PMID: 14505546
[30] Ingram JR, Thomas GA, Rhodes J, Green JT, Hawkes ND, Swift JL, Srivastava ED, Evans BK, Williams GT, Newcombe RG, Courtney E, Pillai S.A randomized trial of nicotine enemas for active ulcerative colitis.Clin Gastroenterol Hepatol. 2005;3(11):1107-14. PMID: 16271342
[31] Leung Y, Panaccione R, Hemmelgarn B, Jones J. Exposing the weaknesses: a systematic review of azathioprine efficacy in ulcerative colitis. Dig Dis Sci. 2008;53(6):1455-61. PMID: 17932752
[32] Khan KJ, Dubinsky MC, Ford AC, Ullman TA, Talley NJ, Moayyedi P. Efficacy of immunosuppressive therapy for inflammatory bowel disease: a systematic review and meta-analysis. Am J Gastroenterol. 2011;106(4):630-42. PubMed PMID: 21407186
[33] Danese S, Angelucci E, Malesci A, Caprilli R.Biological agents for ulcerative colitis: hypes and hopes. Med Res Rev. 2008; 28(2):201-18. PMID: 17464967
[34] Aberra FN, Lichtenstein GR. Infliximab in ulcerative colitis. Gastroenterol Clin North Am. 2006; 35(4): 821-36. PMID: 17129815
[35] Sanchez-Munoz F, Dominguez-Lopez A, Yamamoto-Furusho JK. Role of cytokines in inflammatory bowel disease.World J Gastroenterol. 2008;14(27):4280-8. PMID: 18666314
[36] Fina D, Caruso R, Pallone F, Monteleone G.Interleukin-21 (IL-21) controls inflammatory pathways in the gut. Endocr Metab Immune Disord Drug Targets. 2007;7(4):288-91. PMID: 18220949

[37] Scaldaferri F, Fiocchi C.Inflammatory bowel disease: progress and current concepts of etiopathogenesis.J Dig Dis. 2007;8(4):171-8. PMID: 17970872
[38] Chande N, McDonald JW, Macdonald JK, Wang JJ. Unfractionated or low-molecular weight heparin for induction of remission in ulcerative colitis. Cochrane Database Syst Rev. 2010;(10):CD006774. PubMed PMID: 20927749
[39] Seow CH, Benchimol EI, Griffiths AM, Steinhart AH. Type I interferons for induction of remission in ulcerative colitis. Cochrane Database Syst Rev. 2008;(3):CD006790. PubMed PMID: 18646167
[40] Green JT, Thomas GA, Rhodes J. Nicotine: therapeutic potential for the treatment of ulcerative colitis. Expert Opin Investig Drugs. 1997;6(1):17-22. PMID: 15989558
[41] Xu L. Dr. Dong Demao's experience in treating chronic ulcerative colitis. J Tradit Chin Med. 2004;24(4): 243-6.PMID: 15688686
[42] Chen Q, Zhang H. Clinical study on 118 cases of ulcerative colitis treated by integration of traditional Chinese and Western medicine. J Tradit Chin Med. 1999;19(3):163-5.PMID: 10921142
[43] Zhang X. 23 cases of chronic nonspecific ulcerative colitis treated by acupuncture and moxibustion.J Tradit Chin Med. 1998;18(3):188-91.PMID: 10453610
[44] Wu HG, Yao Y, Shen XY, Tan LY, Shi Y, Yang Y, Liu HR, Zheng S. Comparative study on infrared radiation spectrum of yuan point and Xiahe point of the large intestine channel in the patient of ulcerative colitis.Zhongguo Zhen Jiu. 2008;28(1):49-55.PMID: 18257191
[45] Lee DH, Kim JI, Lee MS, Choi TY, Choi SM, Ernst E. Moxibustion for ulcerative colitis: a systematic review and meta-analysis. BMC Gastroenterol. 2010;10:36. PubMed PMID: 20374658; PubMed Central PMCID: PMC2864201
[46] Roses RE, Rombeau JL.Recent trends in the surgical management of inflammatory bowel isease.World J Gastroenterol. 2008;14(3):408-12. PMID: 18200663
[47] Person B. Laparoscopic surgery for inflammatory bowel diseases.Minerva Chir.2008; 63(2): 151-60. PMID: 18427446
[48] Barnich N, Darfeuille-Michaud A. Role of bacteria in the etiopathogenesis of inflammatory bowel disease.World J Gastroenterol. 2007;13(42):5571-6. PMID: 17948930
[49] Kennedy LD.Nicotine therapy for ulcerative colitis.Ann Pharmacother. 1996;30(9):1022-3.PMID: 8876866
[50] Mannon PJ, Hornung RL, Yang Z, Yi C, Groden C, Friend J, Yao M, Strober W, Fuss IJ. Suppression of inflammation in ulcerative colitis by interferon-β-1a is accompanied by inhibition of IL-13 production. Gut. 2011;60(4):449-55. PubMed PMID: 20971977
[51] Neuman MG.Immune dysfunction in inflammatory bowel disease.Transl Res. 2007;149(4):173-86. PMID: 17383591
[52] Ford AC, Sandborn WJ, Khan KJ, Hanauer SB, Talley NJ, Moayyedi P. Efficacy of biological therapies in inflammatory bowel disease: systematic review and meta-analysis. Am J Gastroenterol. 2011;106(4): 644-59, quiz 660. PubMed PMID: 21407183

4

New Biologic Drugs for Ulcerative Colitis

Francesca Zorzi, Emma Calabrese and Francesco Pallone
Gastrointestinal Unit, Department of Internal Medicine, University of Rome Tor Vergata, Italy

1. Introduction

Inflammatory bowel diseases (IBD) are chronic remittent or progressive inflammatory conditions that may affect the gastrointestinal tract. Crohn's disease (CD) and Ulcerative colitis (UC) are two main phenotypes of IBD. Their etiopathogenesis has not been elucidated but is thought to involve a complex interplay among genetic, environmental, microbial and immune response (1). In the last two decade the advances in our knowledge of the pathogenesis mechanism underlying chronic inflammation in the gut, together with the increase progress in biotechnology have led to the development of a number of biological agent that selectively target specific molecules and pathway involve in gut inflammation. We briefly review the mechanism of action and the efficacy of biological agent in UC.

2. Pathogenetic background

2.2 Genetics factors

Both types of IBD occur in genetically susceptible individuals. IBD, considered a polygenic disorder, is familial in 5-10% and sporadic in the remainder (2). In UC phenotypic concordance in monozygotic twins is less frequent (10-20%) than in CD (50-70%), suggesting that the environmental factors play a more important role. Genetic studies, including genome wide association studies (GWASs) have improved our knowledge on the importance of genetic susceptibility in IBD. Interesting GWASs revealed a substantial overlap in genetic risk factors between CD and UC (3). However it is possible that this similitude is not shared at the level of structurally or functionally relevant polymorphisms. However some loci are quite unique for UC or for CD. For example loci related to regulatory pathways (IL10) intestinal epithelial cell function (ECM1) and HERC2 appear to be specific for UC. A striking outcome of GWASs is that the vast majority of identified loci individually confer a modest risk (odds ratios 1.11 and 1.29). The genetic basis for sporadic IBD may be due to the cumulative effect of interaction of unknown quantities of potentially thousands of common single nucleotide polymorphisms of minor individual biologic impact.

2.3 Environmental factors

The discordance of IBD among monozygotic twins and the development of IBD in immigrants to high prevalence countries and in countries under going rapid Westernization also highlight the importance of environmental factors in disease pathogenesis. Elements within a changing environmental that might affect development of the mucosal immune system and the enteric microflora include improved hygiene, consummation of sterile and no fermented foods, vaccination and age at first exposure to intestinal pathogens (4). The effects of poorly hygiene at early childhood are diverse; in some situation poor hygiene can lead to increase pathogenic infections, but in others it results in a higher exposure to harmless microorganisms and priming of the regulatory immune system, thus lowering the risk for development of IBD. Other environmental factors could affect the disease phenotype is the cigarette smoking that has an opposite effect on the outcome of each form of IBD, most reports have shown that no smoking is a feature of patients in UC, whereas smoking is a feature of CD patients (5-6). A cigarette smoking has been shown to affect cellular ad humoral immunity (7-8), and to increase mucous production (9). Results from in vivo studies have shown that nicotine also has an inhibitory effect on Th2 function that predominates in UC.

2.4 Microbial flora

The contest of the intestinal lumen plays a central role in gut homeostasis. The gastrointestinal tract harbors more than 10^{14} microorganisms of more than 1000 species. Most belong to two different phyla that account for the majority of gram-negative bacteria (bacterioides) and gram-positive bacteria (Firmicutes). Collectively, the microbiota carries out many physiological functions important in mammalian biology. In fact, the microbiota is required for the development and differentiation of local and systemic immune and nonimmune components (10). Systemic immune responses are also impaired in germ-free mice, including the development of adequate Treg responses leading to increased systemic autoimmunity (11), which may have implication for the development of extraintestinal manifestation in IBD. Luminal bacteria appear to provide the stimulus for immuno-inflammatory responses leading to mucosal injury. In IBD mucosal production of IgG antibodies against intestinal bacteria is highly increased, and mucosal defense relies on both IgG mediated responses within the tissue and hyperactivated lymphocytes in the lamina propria reacting against bacterial antigens. These combined events result in inflammation and tissue injury. The altered immune response is not specifically addressed or polarized toward a single group of potential pathogens, but involves a large and undefined number of commensal species belonging to the common enteric flora. Several factors may contribute to the abnormal reactivity of the mucosal immune system against enteric bacteria, and these include genetic susceptibility, a defect in mucosal barrier function, and a microbial imbalance in the gut ecosystem (1).

Several studies have shown that the composition of the fecal microbiota differs between subjects with IBD and healthy controls. The reported differences are variable and not always consistent among the various studies. However, molecular studies show that a substantial proportion of fecal bacteria (up to 30%–40% of dominant species) in patients with active IBD belong to phylogenetic groups that are unusual in healthy subjects (12).

2.5 Immuno-inflammatory factors

This complex interaction of genetic, environment and microbial factors culminates in a sustained activation of the mucosal immune and non immune response resulting in active chronic inflammation and tissue damage (1).

In the healthy gut the mucosal immune system maintains a balance between pro- and anti-inflammatory factors, thereby allowing an effective defense against luminal pathogens while simultaneously preventing an overactive immune response. In IBD, this balance is altered with a shift toward a proinflammatory state owing to a deregulated immune system with a complex interplay between effect and regulatory T cells and immunosuppressive and proinflammatory cytokines (13).

3. Definition of biologic therapy

The promise of biologic therapy is the direct translation of the knowledge of basic mechanisms of disease into therapies of enhanced specificity. Biologic therapies encompass agents of diverse modes of action. Biologic therapies may be considered to fall under five broad categories: (a) native biologic preparations and isolates, included proteins isolated from blood or serum, such as clotting factors or immune globulins, as well as classic vaccines incorporating live, attenuated, or killed microorganisms, or their isolated subunits; (b) recombinant peptides or proteins, many diverse classes of peptides and proteins with the shared feature of having been produced in recombinant cell-based systems, such as bacteria, yeast, or mammalian cells in culture. Most important are recombinant cytokines, cytokine receptor antagonists, and soluble receptors for cytokines and other relevant ligands; (c) antibody-based therapies, monoclonal antibodies may be used for therapeutic purposes, but their utility may be limited by the development of humoral immunity against these non-native proteins; (d) nucleic acid-based therapies, the most promising agents of this type are antisense oligonucleotides. These agents consist of synthetic oligonucleotides of single-stranded DNA bearing a sequence complementary to that of a targeted mRNA species. (e) Cell and gene therapies, include techniques that may alter autologous or donor cell populations. This category may include the treatment of targeted cells with various factors or cytokines ex vivo, or the insertion or deletion of targeted genes in isolated cells ex vivo followed by reintroduction into the host. Alternatively, genetic manipulation may be accomplished by means of viral or plasmid vectors in vivo (14).

4. New biologic drugs for UC

4.1 Blockade of T-cell activation

T cell activation requires two signals. The first signal is mediated by the interaction of the T cell receptor complex, with includes CD4 and CD3, with the antigenic peptides presented by major histocompatibility complex molecules on the surface of antigen presenting cells; the second signals (the costimulatory signals), is antigen non specific and is provided by the interaction between costimulatory molecules expressed on the membrane of antigen presenting cells and the T cell, activation of T cell without costimulatory signals leads to T cell anergy, deletion or immune tolerance.

4.1.1 Anti CD4+ antibodies

Anti CD4 antibodies have been used in a variety of autoimmune disease, and have been tested in CD and UC. A CD4 depleting antibody (cM-T412) was tested in one open label study in UC patients achieved clinical and endoscopic improvement/remission after a period of treatment ranging from seven to eleven days (15). In another three open trials a CD4 no depleting antibodies (MAX.16H5 and B-F5) were administered to nine UC patients with active disease; of the nine patients, five achieved remission. Thus, CD4 depleting antibodies seem to be more effective than no depleting antibodies therapy. However, this specific treatment was most associated with a significant decrease in CD4 cells, and because of concerns of CD4 lynmphopenia no further studies have been performed (16,17).

4.1.2 Anti CD3+ antibodies

Visilizumab (HuM291) is a non-fragment crystallized region (FcR) binding anti CD3 monoclonal antibody directed against invariant CD3ε chain of the T cell receptor; this compound was studied in patients with severe refractory UC. In an open label phase I/II trials, eight patients received a 15 µg/Kg intravenous bolus dose of Visilizumab on two consecutive days and two others received 10 µg/Kg. Remission was achieved after 1 month in seven of the eight patients in the 15 µg/Kg group and after 15 days in all patients in the 10 µg/Kg group. All 8 patients in the high dose group showed improvement based on endoscopic assessment. Endoscopic lesions were absent or only mild in six out of eight patients, and most patients in remission managed to fully taper off their concomitant steroids treatment. An extension of these original trials comprised a total of 24 patients treated with 10 µg/Kg Visilizumab. On day 30 clinical improvement, remission rate and endoscopic remission were observed in 84%, 66% and 44% of patients. After one year, ten out of 22 patients did not require surgical or medical salvage therapy and colectomies were performed for intractable colitis in seven patients during follow up evaluation with a median time to colectomy of 160 days (18). However a phase III randomized double blind placebo controlled multicenter study of Visilizumab in patients with intravenously steroids refractory ulcerative colitis was withdrawn and the Visilizumab was terminated because an interim analysis showed no difference in colectomy rates from Visilizumab versus placebo (19).

4.1.3 Anti IL2-receptor (CD25)

CD25 is a membrane receptor expressed by activated T lymphocytes. IL-2 is a cytokine produced by T cells that induced lymphocyte proliferation and clonally expansion. Cyclosporine, a calcineurin inhibitor, which inhibits IL-2, is effective for the treatment of severely active ulcerative colitis; therefore it was proposed that blocking IL-2 would be an effective therapy for ulcerative colitis (20).

Daclizumab (Zanapax, Protein Designed Labs) is a recombinant humanized IgG1 monoclonal antibody to IL-2 receptor, witch blocks the binding of IL-2 to the receptor (CD25). In an open label pilot trial, ten patients were included and were given two intravenous doses (1 mg/Kg) with 4 weeks interval between doses. Promising response rates at 8 weeks suggested that it was beneficial for patient with active UC (21). Subsequently a randomized double blind placebo control trial was conduced to evaluate the efficacy of induction therapy with Daclizumab in active UC patients. One hundred and nine patients with moderate UC were assigned randomly to groups that were given intravenously 1 mg/Kg dose at weeks 0 and 4; 2 mg/Kg dose at weeks 0,2,4 and 6 compared with patients that received placebo. At week 8 remissions and responses respectively were observed in 2% and 25% of patients receiving Daclizumb 1 mg/Kg and 7% and 33% of patients receiving 2 mg/Kg compared with 10% and 44% of those received placebo. Daclizumab failed to show any efficacy in active UC (22).

Basilizumab (Simulect, Novartis), a chimeric anti CD25 monoclonal IgG1 antibody was evaluated only in open label pilot trial. Fifteen patients received Basilizumab in addition to their standard steroid treatment to evaluate the efficacy of treatment as a steroids sensitizing agent in steroid-resistant UC. Eighty per cent of patients achieved remission within 6 weeks (23). Basilizumab was evaluated only in open label trials and the data might show efficacy but larger placebo controlled trials are needed.

4.1.4 Abadacept

Abatacept modulates naïve T-cell activation and downstream cytokine production. It is a fully human, soluble fusion protein, which consists of the extracellular domain of human cytotoxic T-lymphocyte-associated antigen-4 (CTLA-4) linked to the Fc portion of human immunoglobulin G1. The CTLA-4 portion of the molecule interrupts the CD80/ CD86:CD28 costimulatory signal, mimicking a native homoeostatic mechanism of T-cell down regulation. It is effective in treating patients with rheumatoid arthritis and phase III trials are underway to test its effects in patients with UC and CD.

4.2 Inflammatory cytokines

4.2.1 Anti tumor necrosis factors

TNF-α is a proinflammatory cytokine that has a critical role in the amplification of mucosal inflammation in IBD. TNF-α acts as transmembrane or soluble proteins by transducing signals ranging from cellular activation and proliferation to cytotoxicity and apoptosis through two distinct TNF receptors (TNFR1 and TNFR2). The currently most efficacious treatment for IBD is anti-TNF antibodies. Actually three anti TNF molecules are studied to treat UC.

Infliximab is a monoclonal chimeric antibody, targeting TNF-α composed of a human constant region IgG1K light chain, accounting for approximately 75% of antibody, linked to a mouse variable region (25%). Initially Infliximab did not seem to have much therapeutic effect on UC. Two small pilot trials showed disappointing results for the drug in the treatment of refractory UC (24-25). Recently a new role of Infliximab in the treatment of UC has been offered by two large placebo controlled trials ACT1 and ACT2 (26). In the ACT1 364 patients with active UC with endoscopic evidence of moderate-severe were randomly assigned to receive placebo or Infliximab 5 mg/Kg or 10 mg/Kg at weeks 0, 2, 6 and every 8 weeks through to week 46. At week 8 38,8% patients receiving 5 mg/kg dose and 32% of patients receiving the higher dose achieved remission comparing 14.9% of patients receiving placebo. This difference in remission rates was maintained at week 30 (33.9% 5 mg/kg, 36.9% 10 mg/kg versus 15.7% placebo). Mucosal healing was achieved at weeks 8 and 30 respectively in 62% and 50.4% in the lower dose group, in 59% and 49.2% in the higher dose, and in 33.9% and 24.8% in the placebo group. In the ACT2 study 364 UC patients, refractory to at least one standard therapy were randomly assigned to receive placebo or Infliximab 5 mg/Kg or 10 mg/Kg at weeks 0, 2, 6, 14 and 22. Clinical remission evaluated at week 8 and 30 were respectively 33.9% and 25.6% in 5 mg/kg Infliximab group, 27.5% and 35.8% in 10 mg/Kg Infliximab group versus 5.7% and 10.6% in the placebo group. Mucosal healing was achieved at weeks 8 and 30 respectively in 60.3% and 46.3% in the lower dose group, in 61.7% and 56.7% in the high dose group, and in 30.9% and 30.1% in the placebo group. In both trials Infliximab was well tolerated and induces and maintains clinical response and mucosal healing in moderate to severe UC patients.

Adalimumab is a fully human IgG1 monoclonal antibody to TNF-α that is administrated subcutaneously and easily can be self administrated every 2 weeks. In the first randomized double-blind controlled trial of efficacy and safety of Adalimumab for the induction of clinical remission in 390 patients with moderate to severe active UC (27). Patients were administrated either with placebo or Adalimumab every two weeks for a total of four doses over a 6 week period. Adalimumab was administrated according to one of the following dosage scheduled: 1) 160 mg at week 0, 80 mg at week 2 and 40 mg at week 4 and 6; 2) 80 mg at week 0 and 40 mg at weeks 2,4, and 6. At week 8, 18.5% of patients received Adalimumab 160/80/40 mg had achieved remission (p=0.031 verso placebo), which was significantly greater proportion than those patients received Adalimumab 80/40 mg (10%)(0.833 verso placebo) or placebo (9.2%). No significant differences were observed in the rate of serious adverse events. Adalimumab was therefore well tolerated and effectively induced remission in approximately one-fifth of patients with moderate to severe active UC. In this trial numerous secondary end points were also positive for the higher dose of Adalimumab. Despite the relative poor comparative performance of Adalimumab that, perhaps, suggests inadeguate dosing in the UC trials, several open-label series have reported benefits from Adalimumab in UC patients who responded, but became intolerant of Infliximab. (28,29).

RDP58 is a novel anti-inflammatory decapeptide able to clock TNF production at a post transcriptional step (30) and also inhibits production of IFN-γ, IL-2 and IL-12. RDP58 has been shown to be effective in murine and primate models of colitis (31, 32). In a phase II study 127 patients with mild moderate UC were randomly assigned to receive placebo or an oral solution of RDP58 at 100, 200 or 300 mg daily for 28 days. Clinical remission was achieved in 72% of patients in the 300 mg group, 70% of patients in the 200 mg group and 29% in the lower dose exhalation versus the placebo group. There were any differences in adverse events among treatments group compared to placebo group (33).

4.2.2 Immunomodulators: reconbinant human Interferon α and β

IFNs α and β are produced by virally infected cells and inhibit viral replication within host cells, activate natural killer cells and macrophage, and increase antigen presentation to lymphocytes. IFNs α and β have been investigated in UC with no success. In a multicenter double blind placebo controlled trial, patients with moderate active UC were randomized to receive two doses of INF-β-1a (44 and 66 mcg subcutaneously 3 times weekly for 8 weeks) versus placebo. No differences between INF-β-1a and placebo were observed at 12 weeks (34).

4.3 Anti inflammatory cytokines

IL-10 is an anti-inflammatory cytokine produced by T cells, B cells and monocyte activated lipopolysaccharides. When the body is presented with an antigen, IL-10 inhibits the production of IL-1α, IL-6 and TNF-α. Thus, it contributes to down regulation of acute inflammatory responses (13) In animal models, IL-10 maintains immune homeostasis in the gut and may play a role in the treatment of IBD (35). A phase II placebo-controlled dose response trial with recombinant IL-10 (rHuIL-10) failed to show a beneficial effect in 94 UC patients with mild to severe active disease (36). Development of systemic administration of rHuIL-10 for IBD was discontinued because of lack of efficacy in controlled trials but other animal studies showed that local administration of IL-10 to the colon via genetically engineered *Lactococcus lactis* bacteria that are administered orally allows for the achievement of high colonic mucosal concentration of IL-10, resulting potentially in increased efficacy. It is possible that this approach to IL-10 therapy will be an alternative therapeutic approach for IBD (37).

4.4 Selective adhesion molecule inhibitors

Leukocyte adhesion in high endothelial venules of the gut is a multistep process. Fast moving immune cells are first slowed down by interaction of selectins and non-activated integrins with their respective ligands expressed by endothelial cells. This causes tethering and rolling of leukocytes close to the endothelial surface. Chemokines secreted from sites of inflammation diffuse through the endothelial layer, bind to chemokine receptors and activate integrins. Firm adhesion is the last step before leukocyte diapedesis through endothelial pores and results from strong binding between activated α4β7 integrins with their ligand, mucosal addressing cellular adhesion molecule-1 (38). Agent that block interaction between adhesion molecules on circulating immune cells and their endothelial cell receptors wound be expected to decrease the migration of these cells through the endothelium, thereby decrease chronic inflammation (39).

Natalizumab is a recombinant humanized IgG4 monoclonal antibody to α4 integrin that block adhesion and subsequent leukocyte migration into the gut. It inhibits both α4β7integrin/MAdCAM-1 interaction and α4β7/VCAM-1 binding. Natalizumab 3mg/Kg single intravenous infusion has also demonstrated some evidence of clinical benefit at two weeks post infusion in an uncontrolled study in 10 patients with active UC. Five out of 10 patients achieved a good clinical response at 2 weeks and one more patients at 4 weeks, defined by a Powell-Tuck score of $\leq$ 5 (40). Natalizumab was withdrawn voluntarily from the marked in February 2005 for safety evaluation after one fatal and one non fatal case of progressive multifocal leukoencephalopathy (PML) occurred in the group of 1869 patients who were treated with Natalizumab in combination with Interferon-β-1a over a 2 years period for treatment of multiple sclerosis. Although the 3 case of PML, a review by Youry et al of more than 3000 patients who have received Natalizumab for multiple sclerosis, CD or rheumatoid arthritis suggested a risk of PML of 1/1000 patients treated with Natalizumab for a mean duration of 17.9 months (41). Natalizumab was reintroduced to the market for multiple sclerosis and CD in the United States.

Vedolizumab (formerly MLN-02 and LDP-02) is a humanized anti- α4β7-integrin antibody MLN-0002, that selectively inhibits leukocyte adhesion in the gastrointestinal mucosa. Therefore this compound is being developed only in IBD. A fase I/II, double blind, place controlled, ascending dose trial examined the safety and pharmacology of MLN-0002 in 28 UC patients with moderate severe disease (42). Patients received a single dose of 0.15 mg/kg s.c., a single dose of 0.15, 0.50, or 2.0 mg/kg e.v. or placebo. MLN_0002 appeared to be a generally well-tolerated and effective therapy for active UC. Four years later a multicenter double blind placebo controlled trial was performing involving 181 patients with active UC confirmed efficacy of MLN-0002 in the treatment of active disease. Patients were treated with 2 intravenous dose, 28 days apart, of 0.5 mg/kg or 2.0 mg/Kg of MLN-0002 or placebo. At week 6, clinical remission rates were 33%, 32% and 14% in the groups given 0.5 mg/Kg of MLN-0002, 2.0 mg/kg of MLN-0002 and placebo respectively; percentage of patients who improved by at least 3 points on UC clinical score were respectively 66%, 53% and 33%. Remission was observed by endoscopy in 28% in the lower dose of MLN-0002, in 12% in the higher dose group compared with 8% in the placebo group (43).

The interaction of lymphocyte-associated $\alpha_1\beta_2$-integrin and its ligand ICAM-1 (Intracellular adhesion molecule-1) is important for the recruitment of leukocytes to inflammatory sites. Alicaforsen (ISIS 2302) is a 20-base phosohorothioate antisense oligodeoxynucleotide. It is designed to hybridize to a 3′ untranslated region of human ICAM-1 messenger ribonucleic acid (mRNA). The heterodimer formed is cleaved by ubiquitous ribonuclease H, resulting in a reduction in ICAM-1 protein expression (44). Initial positive results in CD patients reported in a pilot study were not confirmed in two subsequent placebo controlled trial (45-47). Instead in a placebo controlled trial with ISIS 2302 in enema formulation showed significant improvement in 40 patients with distal UC (48). In a phase 2, dose-ranging, double-blind, placebo-controlled study, 112 patients with mild-moderate left-sided UC received one of four ISIS 2302 enema regimens or placebo daily for 6 weeks (49). While there were no significant differences between treatment or placebo in terms of DAI at week 6, there was a prolonged reduction in the mean percentage DAI relative to baseline from week 18 (51% versus 18% p=0.04) to week 30 (50% versus 11% p=0.03) in the 240 mg ISIS 2302 group compared with placebo.

Monoclonal antibodies to Madcam-1 and integrin β7 subunit (50) are currently being tested in clinical trials..

4.5 Growth factors

Epithelial growth factors are naturally occurring proteins capable of stimulating cellular growth, proliferation and differentiation. A potent mitogenic peptide produced by salivary glands, epidermal growth factors (EGF) and keratinocyte growth factor (KGF) may play an important role in IBD for their potential use to restore mucosal integrity (51). In UC the inflammation is confined to the mucosa and epithelial cell damage is an important feature.

Repifermin (KGF-2) has been shown to reduce inflammation in animal models of colitis (52-54). The effect of Repifermin were studied in a phase II, placebo controlled trial in 88 patients with active UC. Patients were randomized to receive treatment for five consecutive days with intravenous repifermin at a dose of 1, 5, 10, 25 or 50 lg/kg, or placebo. Intravenous repifermin at a dose of 1–50 µg/kg was very well tolerated, but there was no evidence that repifermin was effective for the treatment of active UC at these doses (55).

In randomized, double-blind clinical trial conducted, 12 patients with mild-to-moderate left-sided UC received daily enemas of 5 µg of EGF in 100 ml of an inert carrier and 12 patients received daily enemas with carrier alone for 14 days, all patients also began to receive 1.2 gr of oral mesalamine per day or had their dose increased by 1.2 gr per day. After two weeks, 10 of the 12 patients treated with EGF enemas were in remission, as compared with 1 of 12 in the control group (83 percent vs. 8 percent, P<0.001). At the 2-week assessment, disease-activity score, endoscopic score and histology score were all significantly better in the EGF group than in the placebo group (p<0.01 for all comparisons), and this benefit was maintained at 4 and at 12 weeks. This study provides preliminary data suggesting that EGF enemas are an effective treatment for active left-sided UC (56). Further studies are warranted, but the safety of therapy stimulating EGF in UC is most importantly because it up regulates the expression of protoncogen in patients with known colon cancer risk.

5. Conclusion: The state of art biologic agent in UC

Over the last two decades, advances in bio-technology together with the increasing knowledge about the pathogenesis of IBD and the mechanism driving the uncontrolled inflammation led to discovery new targets for a large number of biological agents. The improved understanding of pathogenic mechanisms and the basis of heterogeneity within the disease group should lead to different therapeutic approaches for various disease phenotypes and eventually to personalize treatment. The benefits for anti-TNF therapy in UC have opened the door of clinical practice for additional anti-TNF or for agents with alternative targets. Early studies have suggested potential benefits of inhibiting adhesion molecules such as α4β7 integrins or inhibition of ICAM-1; on the other hand studies evaluating therapies targeting T cell activation have been disappointing. Finally, given that the efficacy, short-term and long term for the newer biological therapeutics are either limited or remain to be proven on a large number of patients, the use of such agents in patients remains to be estimated and tailored on the single patient.

6. References

[1] Kaser A, Zeissing S, Blumberg RS. Inflammatory Bowel Disease. Annu Rev Immunol. 2010;28:573-621.

[2] Halme L, Paavola-Sakki P, Turunen U, et al. Family and twin studies in inflammatory bowel disease. World J. Gastroenterol. 2006;12:3668-72.

[3] Budarf ML, Labbe C, David G, et al. GWA studies: rewriting the story of IBD. Trends Genet. 2009;25:137-46.

[4] Shanahnan F. Crohn's Disease. Lancet. 2002;359:62-69.

[5] Franceschi S, Panza E, La vecchia C, et al. Non specific inflammatory bowel disease and smoking. Am J Epidemiol. 1987;125:445-452.

[6] Linberg E, Tysk C, Anderson K, et al. Smoking and Inflammatory bowel disease: a case control study. Gut. 1988;29:252-357.

[7] Miller LG, Goldstein G, Murphy M, et al. Reversible alteration in immunoregulatory T cells in smoking: analysis by monoclonal antibodies and flow cytometry. Chest.1982;82:526-529.

[8] Srivastava ED, Barton JR, O'Mahony S. Smoking, humoral immunity, and ulcerative colitis. Gut. 1991;32:1016-1019.

[9] Cope GF, Heatley RV, Kelleher JK. Smoking and colonic mucous in ulcerative colitis. BMJ. 1986;293:481.

[10] Round JL, Mazmanian SK. The gut microbiota shapes intestinal immune responses during health amd diseaseNat Rev Immunol. 2009X

[11] Mazmanian SK, Round JL, Kasper DL. Amicrobial symbiosis factor prevents intestinal inflammatory disease. Nature. 2008;453:620-625

[12] Ott SJ, Musfeld M, Wenderoth DF, et al. Reduction in diversity of the colonic mucosa associated bacterial microflora in patients with active inflammatory bowel disease. Gut 2004;53:658-693

[13] Izcue A, Coombes JL, Powrie F. Regulatory Lymphocytes and Intestinal Inflammation. Annu Rev Immunol. 2009;27:313-338.

[14] Sands BE. Biologic therapy for inflammatory bowel disease. Inflamm Bowel Dis. 1997;3:95-113.

[15] Deusch K, Mauthe B, Reiter C, et al. CDA-antibody treatment of inflammatory bowel disease: one year follow-up. Gastroenterology. 1993;104:A691
[16] Emmrich J, Seyfarth M, Fleig WE, et al. Treatment of inflammatory bowel disease with anti-CD4 monoclonal antibody. Lancet 1991; 338:570-571
[17] Emmrich J, Seyfarth M, Liebe S, et al. Anti-CD6 antibody treatment in inflammatory bowel disease without a long $CD4^{+}$-cell depletion. Gastroenterology. 1995;108:A815.
[18] Plevy SE, Salzberg BA, Van Assche G, et al. A phase I study of visilizuma, a humanized anti-CD3 monoclonal antibody, for treatment of severe steroid-refractory ulcerative colitis. Gastroenterology.2007;133:1414-1422.
[19] Sandborn WJ, Colombel JF, Frankel M, et al. Anti CD3-antibody visilizumab is not effective in patients with intravenous corticosteroid-refractory ulcerative colitis. Gut. 2010; Nov;59(11):1485-92.
[20] Van Assche G, D'Haens G, Noman M, et al. Randomized, double-blind comparison of 4 mg/kg versus 2 mg/kg intravenous cyclosporine in severe ulcerative colitis. Gastroenterology 2003;125(4):1025-31.
[21] Van Assche G, Dalle I, Noman M, et al. Apilot study on the use of the ulcerative colitis. Am J Gastroenterol. 2003; 98:369-376.
[22] Van Assche G, Sandborn WJ, Feagan BG, et al. Daclizumab, a humanised monoclonal antibody to the interleukin 2 receptor (CD25), for the treatment of moderately to severely active ulcerative colitis: a randomised, double blind, placebo-controlled, dose ranging trial. Gut. 2006;55:1568–1574.
[23] Creed TJ, Norman MR, Probert CS, et al. Basiliximab (anti-CD25) in combination with steroids may be an effective new treatment for steroid-resistant ulcerative colitis. Aliment Pharmacol Ther. 2003;18:1865–1875.
[24] Chey WY, Hussain A, Ryan C, et al. Infliximab for refractory ulcerative colitis. Am J Gastroenterol. 2001;96:2373–2381.
[25] Sands BE, Tremaine WJ, Sandborn WJ, et al. Infliximab in the treatment of severe, steroid-refractory ulcerative colitis: a pilot study. Inflamm Bowel Dis. 2001;7:83–88.
[26] Rutgeerts P, Sandborn WJ, Feagan BG, et al. Infliximab for induction and maintenance therapy for ulcerative colitis. N Engl J Med. 2005;353:2462–2476.
[27] Reinisch W, Sandborn WJ, Hommes DW, et al. Adalimumab for induction of clinical remission in moderately to severely active ulcerative colitis. Gut. 2011; 60:780-787.
[28] Afif W, Leighton JA, Hanauer SB, et al.. Open-label study of adalimumab in patients with ulcerative colitis including those with prior loss of response or intolerance to infliximab. Inflammatory Bowel Dis. 2009; 15:1302-1307
[29] Oussalah A, Laclotte C, Chevaux JB, et al. Long-term outcome of adalimumab therapy for ulcerative colitis with intolerance or lost of response to infliximab: a single-centre experience. Aliment Pharmacol Ther 2008; 28:966-972.
[30] Iyer S, Kontoyannis D, Chevrier D, et al. Inhibition of tumor necrosis factor mRNA translation by a rationally designed immunomodulatory peptide. J Biol Chem. 2000;275:17051–17057.
[31] Murthy S, Flanigan A, Coppola D, et al. RDP58, a locally active TNF inhibitor, is effective in the dextran sulphate mouse model of chronic colitis. Inflamm Res. 2002;51:522–531.

[32] Bourreille A, Doubremelle M, de la Bletiere DR, et al. RDP58, a novel immunomodulatory peptide with anti-inflammatory effects. A pharmacological study in trinitrobenzene sulphonic acid colitis and Crohn's disease. Scand J Gastroenetrol. 2003;38:526–532.
[33] Travis SPL, Yap LM, Hawkey CJ, et al. RDP-58: novel and effective therapy, for ulcerative coltis: results of parallel, prospective, placebo- controlled trial. Am J Gastroenterol. 2003;98:S239.
[34] Pena-Rossi C, Schreiber S, Golubovic G, et al. Clinical trial: a multicenter, randomized, double-blind, placebo-controlled, dose-finding, phase II study of subcutaneous interferon-beta-1a in moderately active ulcerative colitis. Aliment Pharmacol Ther. 2008;28:758-767.
[35] Kuhn R, Lohler J, Rennick D, et al. Interleukin-10-deficient mice develop chronic enterocolitis. Cell. 1993;75:263–274
[36] Schreiber S, Fedorak NR, Wild G, et al. Ulcerative Colitis IL-10 Cooperative Study Group. Safety and tolerance of rHuIL-10 treat- ment in patients with mild/moderate active ulcerative colitis. Gastroenterology. 1998;114:A1080–A1081.
[37] Steidler L, Hans W, Schotte L, et al. Treatment of murine colitis by Lactococcus lactis secreting interleukin-10. Science. 2000;289:1352–1355.
[38] Butcher EC, Picker LJ. Lymphocyte homing and homeostasis. Science. 1996;272:60-66.
[39] Sandbirn WJ, Yednock TA. Novel approaches to treating inflammatory bowel disease: targeting alpha-4 integrin: Am J Gastroenterol. 2003; 98:2372-2382.
[40] Gordon FH, Hamilton MI, Donoghue S, et al. A pilot study of treatment of active ulcerative colitis with natalizumab, a humanized monoclonal anti- body to alpha-4 integrin. Aliment Pharmacol Ther. 2002;16:699–705.
[41] Yousry TA, Major EO, Ryschkewitsch C, et al. Evaluation of patients treated with natalizumab for progressive multifocal leukoencephalopathy. N Engl J Med 2006; 354:924-933.
[42] Feagan BC, McDonald J, Greenberg G, et al. An ascending dose trial of a humanized A4B7 antibody in ulcerative colitis (UC). Gastroenterology. 2001;118:A874.
[43] Feagan BG, Greenberg GR, Wild G, et al. Treatment of ulcerative colitis with a humanized antibody to the alpha4beta7 integrin. N Engl J Med. 2005;352:2499-2507.
[44] Bennet CF, Condon TP, Grimm S, et al. Inhibition of endothelial cell adhesion molecule expression with antisense oligonucleotides. J Immunol. 1994;152:3530–3540.
[45] Yacyshyn BR, Bowen-Yacyshyn MB, et al. A placebo- controlled trial of ICAM-1 antisense oligonucleotide in the treatment of Crohn's disease. Gastroenterology. 1998;114:113–142.
[46] Schreiber S, Nikolaus S, Malchow H, et al. Absence of efficacy of subcutaneous antisense ICAM-1 treatment of chronic active Crohn's disease. Gastroenterology. 2001;120:1339–1346.
[47] Yacyshyn BR, Chey WY, Goff J, et al. Double-blind, placebo con- trolled trial of the remission inducing and steroid sparing properties of an ICAM-1 antisense oligodeoxynucleotide, alicaforsen (ISIS 2302), in active steroid dependent Crohn's disease. Gut. 2002;51:30–36.
[48] Van Deventer SJ, Tami JA, Wedel MK. A randomised, controlled, double-bind, escalating dose study of alicaforsen enema in ulcerative colitis. Gut. 2004;53:1646–1651.

[49] Van Deventer SJH, wedel MK, Baker BF et al.A phase II dose ranging, double-blind, placebo-controlled study of alicarforsen enema in subjects with acute exacerbation of mild to moderate left-sided ulcerative colitis. Aliment Pharmacol Ther. 2006;23:1415-1425.
[50] Rutgeerts P, Fedorak R, Daniel W, et al. A Phase I Study of rHuMab Beta7 in Moderate to Severe Ulcerative Colitis (UC). Gastroenterology 2011; 140: A748.
[51] Beck PL, Podolsky DK. Growth factors in inflammatory bowel disease. Inflamm Bowel Dis. 1999;5:44–60.
[52] Sung C, Parry T, Riccobene T, et al. Pharmacologic and pharmacokinetic profile of repifermin (KGF-2) in monkeys and comparative pharmacokinetics in humans. AAPS Pharmsci 2002; 4(2): 1–10.
[53] Han DS, Li F, Holt L, et al. Keratinocyte growth factor-2 (FGF- 10) promotes healing of experimental small intestinal ulcer- ation in rats. Am J Physiol Gastrointest Liver Physiol 2000; 279(5): G1011–22.
[54] Miceli R, Hubert M, Santiago G, et al. Efficacy of keratinocyte growth factor-2 in dextran sulfate sodium-induced murine colitis. J Pharmacol Exp Ther 1999; 290(1): 464–71.
[55] Sandborn WJ, Sands BE, Wolf DC, et al Repifermin (Keratinocyte growth factor-2) for the treatment of active ulcerative colitis: a randomized, double-blind, placebo-controlled, dose-escalation trial. Aliment Pharmacol Ther 2003;17: 1355-1364.
[56] Sinha A, Nightingale J, West KP, et al. Epidermal growth factor enemas with oral mesalamine for mild-to-moderate left-sided ulcerative colitis or proctitis. N Engl J Med. 2003;349:350-357.

5

Clinical, Biological, and Laboratory Parameters as Predictors of Severity of Clinical Outcome and Response to Anti–TNF–Alpha Treatment in Ulcerative Colitis

Trine Olsen and Jon Florholmen
Research group of Gastroenterology and Nutrition, Institute of Clinical Medicine, University of Tromsø, Tromsø and Department of Medical Gastroenterology, University Hospital North Norway, Tromsø, Norway

1. Introduction

Ulcerative colitis (UC) is a chronic relapsing inflammatory bowel disease (IBD). The pathogenesis of IBD is complex and so far not fully understood. The long-term clinical outcome of UC is hard to predict. Some clinical phenotypes of UC may to some extent predict the severity of the disease, but the clinical impact of these predictors is minor. . The new immunomolecular understanding of the pathophysiological mechanisms behind the disease, and especially the genetic engineering knock out animal models in early 1990's, was the start of a new therapeutic strategy: the targeting therapy. Based on new knowledge of proinflammatory and anti-inflammatory molecules, new therapeutic targets were established to attack specific components of the inflammatory cascade. TNF-alpha was the first molecule to be blocked with effects on the disease activity first described in the animal models and then described in humans in 1995 for Crohns disease (CD). Later on, numerous other targeting molecules have been developed with more or less efficacy. So far the anti-TNF agent infliximab (IFX) is the only targeting agent that has been found to be effective in UC. However, a lot still needs to be done in order to achieve "personalized engineered therapy" in IBD. After some ten years experiences with targeting therapy the major unresolved questions are: which UC patients will have the greatest effect of targeting therapy inducing a "deep, longstanding" remission and prevent severe outcome such as colectomy? Which patients are in the need of long-term maintenance therapy? If and when can target therapy be stopped? Few studies have investigated potential predictors of the disease's severity and future clinical outcome after the introduction of targeting therapy. Therefore, after ten years with targeting therapy of UC, what clinical, biological or histological markers could give some answers to these questions addressed above?

2. Clinical markers in various clinical settings

Definition of a biological marker

Biomarker is defined by National Institute of health (NIH) as "a characteristic that is objectively measured and evaluated as an indicator of normal biological processes, pathogenic processes, or pharmacological responses to a therapeutic intervention" (Colburn, 2000). An optimal biomarker has to fit into several criteria to be of clinical value. It has to be accurate, reproducibly, acceptable for the patient, and have high sensitivity and specificity for the outcome it is expected to identify (Mendoza and Abreu, 2009). A **prognostic biomarker** should indicate future severe clinical outcomes such as intestinal stenosis and need of surgical resections. This would give valuable information such as priority of treatment options and closer follow-up visits. A **predictive biomarker** should give information of therapeutic effect of agents such as targeting therapy. The ideal biomarker assay from tissue or body fluids should be accurate, reproducible with high sensitivity and specificity. The biomarker concept is old. Despite this, there is a lack of validation of new candidate biomarkers in order to give a useful guidance to the clinicians (2010).

So far no ideal biomarkers have been found in IBD, but several serological and fecal biomarker candidates have been proposed (Mendoza and Abreu, 2009). A biomarker in IBD should predict: the clinical outcome with special emphasis of patients with complicated disease; which therapeutically strategy should be used and especially which patients would be suitable for the high cost treatment of targeting agents; and finally are there biomarkers of resistance to therapy.

In this review we present the candidate biomarkers based on "old", established methods easily performed in a clinical setting, and biomarkers from the new era of high technological methods.

2.1 Demographic factors (clinical phenotypes) as predictors of disease severity and response of treatment

2.1.1 Smoking, age and early onset of disease

In a retrospective study of Roth et al (Roth *et al.*, 2010) one hundred and two UC patients were investigated. In this study charts were reviewed using standardized data collection forms. Disease severity was generated during the chart review process, and non-endoscopic Mayo Score criteria were collected into a composite. They found that UC severity was associated with younger age at diagnosis and year of diagnosis. Previous studies have shown that patients with early onset UC are more prone to colorectal cancer (Eaden *et al.*, 2001). In the study of Roth et al (Roth *et al.*, 2010) disease severity at presentation did not correlate with the severity index over the disease course, nor did delay from diagnosis to treatment. This is in contrast to the literature presented in a review article by Sandborn (Sandborn, 1999) who found that classifying presentations into one of four severity categories was useful for prognosticating disease. Another intriguing result of the study by Roth et al was that smoking status did not predict disease severity (Roth *et al.*, 2010). Multiple previous studies have found that smoking is a protective factor (Calkins, 1989), while non- or ex-smokers have a higher risk of relapsing disease (Hoie *et al.*, 2007). The limitations of the study by Roth et al are that it is retrospective in design and relies heavily on chart review.

2.1.2 ANCAs and ASCA

Perinuclear anti-neutrophil antibody (ANCAs) is associated with chronic inflammatory diseases as Wegener`s granulomatosis, rheumatoid arthritis and UC (Mendoza and Abreu, 2009). In CD the seroprevalence of ANCA ranges from 2-28% and in UC 20-85% (Mendoza and Abreu, 2009). The sensitivity and specificity in diagnosing IBD range from 50-70% and 80-85%, respectively (Mendoza and Abreu, 2009). Anti-saccharomyces cerevisiae antibodies (ASCA) are found in 39%-69% of CD patients, but only in 5-15% of UC patients (Mendoza and Abreu, 2009). The sensitivity and specificity in diagnosing IBD range from 65-70% and 80-85%, respectively (Mendoza and Abreu, 2009).

The clinical value of ANCA or ASCA to differentiate IBD from IBS patients is limited because of low sensitivity. Serologic evaluation of ANCAs and ASCAs may be helpful in patients with indeterminate colitis (Joossens *et al.*, 2002). Interestingly, pANCA in CD patients have been negatively associated with small small bowel disease, fibrostenosis and small bowel surgery (Vermeire *et al.*, 2004), while ASCAs have been associated with several CD clinical phenotypes (Vermeire *et al.*, 2001;Walker *et al.*, 2004). Further, ASCAS have been associated with small bowel disease in CD in addition to stricturing as well as penetrating disease behavior (Mow *et al.*, 2004; Vermeire *et al.*, 2001; Walker *et al.*, 2004). There is also found a strong association between development of pouchitis and high level of ANCAs (Fleshner *et al.*, 2001; Vernier *et al.*, 2004). Though, this has not been confirmed in another study (Aisenberg *et al.*, 2004).

2.2 Biochemical factors reflecting disease activity or responses to specific therapies (C-reactive protein, calprotectin)

2.2.1 C-reactive protein

2.2.1.1 CRP production in ulcerative colitis and Crohn´s disease

C-reactive protein (CRP) is an acute phase protein that increases during inflammation and has a short half life (19 hours) and will therefore rapidly decrease after resolution of the inflammation (Vermeire *et al.*, 2006). Serum CRP as a biomarker in the course of UC has been studied by number of workers but its usefulness as a diagnostic screening test has not been fully assessed. However, CRP is the most sensitive screening biomarker compared to other biomarkers in adult population for detecting IBD, where CD has the strongest CRP response of the two diseases (Lewis, 2011; Vermeire *et al.*, 2006). The reason for this difference between the two diseases is not known. Both CD patients and UC patients have increased levels of cytokines belonging to T-helper-1 response (Olsen *et al.*, 2007; Vermeire *et al.*, 2006). Santos et al investigated 957 subjects and found strong association between CRP and central abdominal obesity (Santos *et al.*, 2005). Positive association between BMI and CRP has also been observed in otherwise healthy adults and children, suggesting a state of low-grade systemic inflammation in obese persons (Visser *et al.*, 1999; Visser *et al.*, 2001). Several groups have investigated adipose tissue and concluded that invasion of inflammatory cells in adipose tissue leads to increased levels of various pro-inflammatory cytokines including IL-6, IL-8, TNF-alpha, IL-10 and IL-18, potentially linking fat and inflammation (Fantuzzi, 2005;Isakson *et al.*, 2009). It has been speculated whether the transmural inflammation in CD and possible involvement of mesenteric fat which is a major site of IL-6 and TNF-alpha synthesis may explain the difference of the two diseases. Colombel et al examined whether small bowel inflammation at CT enterography correlated with endoscopic severity and CRP in 143 patients with CD (Colombel *et al.*, 2006). They concluded that CRP correlated with radiological findings of perienteric inflammation (increased fat density), but not of inflammation limited to the small bowel wall, underscoring the potential role of perienteric inflammation in CRP response in CD. Solem et al confirmed this finding in a recent study where abnormal small bowel radiographic imaging was not associated with CRP elevation in CD patients (Solem *et al.*, 2005). The final conclusions concerning the difference of CRP in UC and CD patients are still not drawn. However, even though the CRP response is strongest in CD, the overlap between CD and UC patients in CRP levels make it difficult to use it for differential diagnosis between the two diseases.

2.2.2 CRP, genetic factors and IBD

Individual genetic factors may also contribute to differences of CRP levels. Recent studies have suggested that polymorphisms in the CRP gene account for the inter-individual differences in baseline CRP production in humans (Carlson *et al.*, 2005) but so far results are conflicting (Vermeire *et al.*, 2006). Interestingly, Greenfield et al investigated 194 healthy female twins to examine the relationship between CRP, BMI, blood pressure, lipids and apolipoproteins, independent of genetic influences (Greenfield *et al.*, 2004). They concluded that CRP was strongly related to total and central abdominal obesity, blood pressure and lipid levels independent of genetic influences (Greenfield *et al.*, 2004).

2.2.3 CRP and the role in predicting disease activity in IBD

In a study by Prantera et al (Prantera *et al.*, 1988) 60 UC patients were investigated and they found that the disease severity and the presence of signs and symptoms of toxicity seemed likely to be determined by the amount of colonic tissue involved by inflammation, both in depth and in extent. CRP appeared the most reliable factor reflecting activity and extension of lesion. In a study from Mayo Clinic (Solem *et al.*, 2005), 43 UC patients were investigated. In this study they concluded that serum CRP levels were associated with increase in biomarkers of inflammation (except platelets) and an active disease at ileocolonoscopy. However, histological activity was not associated with CRP concentrations in UC patients. These results should though be interpreted with caution given the relatively small sample size of 43. In another study Chouhan et al. (Chouhan *et al.*, 2006) concluded that measurement of CRP levels is a simple method of assessing disease activity and extent in UC. They concluded that CRP level >12 mg/L is indicative of severe and extensive disease and that a change in CRP following therapy is a good parameter to assess the effect of the drug on the underlying inflammation. A decrease in CRP in response to therapy is objective evidence that the drug has a beneficial effect on gut inflammation even in patients with little change in symptoms. On the other hand, persistently raised CRP indicates failure of the therapy to control mucosal inflammation (Pepys and Hirschfield, 2003).

In an interesting newly published prospective study of Henriksen et al (Henriksen *et al.*, 2008) CRP was measured at diagnosis and after 1 and 5 years in patients diagnosed with IBD in southeastern Norway. After 5 years, 454 patients with UC and 200 with CD provided sufficient data for analysis. The authors concluded in line with earlier findings that patients with CD had a stronger CRP response than those with UC. In patients with UC, CRP levels at diagnosis increased with increasing extent of disease. However, in this study 71% of patients with UC still had CRP levels within the normal range and mean CRP values were within the normal range in all UC subgroups at 5 years. Further they found that in patients with UC with extensive colitis, CRP levels above 23 mg/l at diagnosis predicted an increased risk of surgery (odds ratio (OR) 4.8, p=0.02). In patients with ulcerative colitis, CRP levels above 10 mg/l after 1 year predicted an increased risk of surgery during the subsequent 4 years (OR 3.0, p=0.02). Interestingly, five years later the authors found no difference in CRP levels between 195 patients who underwent colonoscopy and were in endoscopic remission and those with endoscopic inflammation (mean 6 mg/l versus 7 mg/l, p=0.59). This finding is somehow in contrast to the results of increasing extent of UC correlates with increasing CRP levels. The authors conclude that the results may indicate that CRP is of limited value in predicting disease activity during follow-up. The strength of this Norwegian study is that it is prospective in design (Henriksen *et al.*, 2008). In addition the size of the Norwegian study population seems to be appropriate, in contrast to the study from Mayo Clinic. A minor limitation of the Norwegian study is that it is a multicenter study with different clinicians and therefore there may be some grade of inter-observer variations.

2.2.4 CRP and the role in predicting response to therapy

Several clinical studies have investigated the role of CRP for monitoring the effect of treatment. A decrease in CRP in response to therapy could be objective evidence that the drug has a beneficial effect on gut inflammation. In a recent published Cochrane analysis, the authors included all the randomized controlled trials comparing natalizumab to a placebo or control therapy for the induction of remission in CD (Macdonald and McDonald, 2007). Subgroup analyses demonstrated statistically significant differences in clinical response at twelve weeks favoring three infusions of natalizumab (4 mg/kg) over placebo for CD patients with an elevated CRP at baseline (Macdonald and McDonald, 2007). In a Belgian study 153 CD patients were included and treated with infliximab. Baseline CRP>5 mg/l before the start of therapy was associated with a higher response (76%) compared with patients with CRP<5 mg/l (46%). In line with the findings above, Schreiber et al investigated the efficacy of certolizumab in 292 CD patients and concluded that in the subgroup of patients with low CRP the placebo response rates were high (Schreiber *et al.*, 2005). The situation in UC is more unclear since most of the studies performed concerning CRP and prediction of response to anti-TNF-alpha treatment are done on CD patients (Mendoza and Abreu, 2009; Vermeire *et al.*, 2006). However, Ferrante et al investigated predictors of early response to infliximab in 100 patients with UC (Ferrante *et al.*, 2007). They concluded that pANCA+/ASCA- serotype and an older age at first infliximab infusion were associated with a suboptimal early clinical response, while CRP ≥5 was not a significant predictor (Ferrante *et al.*, 2007). Other studies are done concerning which patients are most likely to respond to intravenous corticosteroid therapy for UC. Travis et al demonstrated that after three days intensive treatment with intravenous steroids, patients with frequent stools (> 8/day), or raised CRP (> 45 mg/l) needed to be identified, as most would require colectomy (Travis *et al.*, 1996). However, clinical scores which is based on symptoms are in some studies found to more accurately identify UC patients who do not respond to intravenous corticosteroids than CRP (Turner *et al.*, 2010).

2.2.5 Summary

Taken together, most of the clinical studies conclude that the values of CRP as a marker in detecting IBD range between 50-60% for UC and between 70-100% for CD and of course depend on the cut off value used (Lewis, 2011;Vermeire *et al.*, 2006). Several study results point in the direction that CRP levels increase with increasing clinical activity of UC. Still it is important to keep in mind that many of the IBD patients have CRP levels within the normal range at diagnosis and this means that measuring CRP does not necessarily differentiate between IBD and functional order (Henriksen *et al.*, 2008;Lewis, 2011). In one Norwegian study CRP levels above 10 mg/l was a predictor of surgery in a subgroup of patients with UC, however few patients with UC underwent surgery in the study and the data should therefore be interpreted with caution. There are also conflicting results in the different studies concerning the correlation between CRP and endoscopic inflammation in UC and CRP and histological inflammation in UC. Further, in CD, a decrease in CRP levels in response to therapy is objective evidence that the drug has a beneficial effect on gut inflammation (Vermeire *et al.*, 2006). In UC the correlation between CRP levels and benefit of treatment is less clear. In conclusion, further studies should be carried out to evaluate whether highly sensitive CRP assays are more sensitive markers of gut inflammation and disease outcome in IBD patients. The conflicting study results concerning endoscopic inflammation and histological inflammation and CRP underscore the fact that measuring CRP in serum is an indirect marker of an inflammation mainly located in the gut and therefore not an optimal biomarker.

2.3 Calprotectin

2.3.1 Introduction

Calprotectin is a protein that removes 60% of the calprotectin protein from the cytosol (Lundberg *et al.*, 2005). Since the first assay was introduced on the market, there has been a change related to the introduction of a new extraction buffer that gives a fivefold better yield of calprotectin during the extraction procedure (Ton *et al.*, 2000). The concentration of calprotectin in feces is an indirect measure of neutrophils infiltrate in the bowel mucosa (Lewis, 2011). Fecal calprotectin levels fluctuate during the course of IBD, but it is well documented that it is persistently elevated during the disease relapse in both adults and children (Berni et al, 2004, Tibble et al, 2000 and 2001). However, calprotectin is not a specific marker. Increased levels are found in other diseases than inflammatory bowel disease, as in colorectal neoplasia, microscopic colitis, food allergy, active celiac disease, allergic colitis, cystic fibrosis, infection and polyps (Carroccio *et al.*, 2003; Tibble *et al.*, 2000a; van Rheenen *et al.*, 2010). It is also found to increase after use of non-steroidal anti-inflammatory drugs, proton pump inhibitor and with increasing age (Carroccio *et al.*, 2003; Tibble *et al.*, 1999; van Rheenen *et al.*, 2010).

2.3.2 Calprotectin as a tool to differentiate IBD from IBS patients

Several studies have been performed investigating the sensitivity and specificity of calprotecting in various clinical settings. In a meta-analysis study by von Roon et al, data from 30 studies was summarized, including 1210 IBD patients, to address whether fecal calprotectin could be used to differentiate IBS patients from IBD patients (von Roon *et al.*, 2007). The calculated sensitivity and specificity values were 0.95 and 0.91 respectively. The diagnostic precision of calprotectin for IBD was higher in children than adults. The fecal calprotectin threshold used in these studies was 50 microgram/gram (von Roon *et al.*, 2007). In another summary by Gisbert et al, 14 different studies were compared (Gisbert *et al.*, 2009). They summarized that the calprotectin sensitivity range from 63-100% and the specificity from 74-98% for the diagnosis of IBD , calculating mean sensitivity and specificity of 80% (95% CI, 77-82%) and 76% (95% CI, 72-79) (Gisbert *et al.*, 2009). In a recent meta-analysis by van Rheenen et al 13 studies were included, six in adults and seven in children and teenagers (van Rheenen *et al.*, 2010). In the studies of adults, the pooled sensitivity and pooled specificity of calprotectin was 0.93 (95% confidence interval 0.85 to0.97) and 0.96 (0.79 to 0.99) and in the studies of children and teenagers was 0.92 (0.84to 0.96) and 0.76 (0.62 to 0.86). The lower specificity in the studies of children and teenagers was significantly different from that in the studies of adults (p=0.048). All three meta-analysis studies concluded that fecal calprotectin has a good diagnostic precision for separating organic and functional intestinal diseases and is a useful screening tool for identifying patients who need endoscopy for suspected IBD. However, the specificity of calprotectin was significant lower in children and teenagers compared to adults in the meta-analysis by van Rheenen, while in the study by von Roon the opposite result was found.

There is a notably variation in the range in both pooled sensitivity and specificity in the different studies summarized in meta-analysis studies, worthwhile to discuss. There may be several explanations for these variations. When comparing different studies one must ensure that the patient populations for each of the two disease states are equivalent and that the study designs are comparable. In the study by Costa et al for example 71% of CD patients had small intestinal disease alone, with only 31% having colitis (Costa *et al.*, 2005). These values are compared with 47% and 53%, respectively, in another study included in the summary (Tibble *et al.*, 2000a). Thus there may be a possible selection bias influencing the final predicative values. Further, the disease activity in most of the studies was assessed by the Crohn's disease activity index (CDAI), a test that is highly subjective and correlates poorly with inflammatory activity assessed by In111 labelled white cells and endoscopic indices (Saverymuttu, 1986). Finally the calprotectin assay has been changed (Ton *et al.*, 2000) in the period of the performed studies summarized by Gisbert et al (Gisbert *et al.*, 2009). In this summary 10/14 studies have used the new and more sensitive calprotectin assay and that may have influenced the final results, as commented by the authors (Gisbert *et al.*, 2009). In the meta-analysis by van Rheenen et al the study quality was assessed using the QUADAS (quality assessment of studies of diagnostic accuracy included in systematic reviews) checklist and from this checklist they chose seven best differentiating items (van Rheenen *et al.*, 2010). The other meta-analysis studies did not select studies in the same way and this may of course influence the difference in the pooled sensitivity and specificity values (Gisbert *et al.*, 2009; von Roon *et al.*, 2007). In addition, von Roon et al pooled the sensitivity and specificity separately contrary to general recommendations and included studies that featured a control group with healthy people, which leads to overestimation of diagnostic accuracy (van Rheenen *et al.*, 2010; von Roon *et al.*, 2007). The pooled sensitivity and specificity in meta-analysis should be interpreted with caution because of the heterogeneity in the different studies included. In summary, the final range of the sensitivity and specificity of calprotectin is still not settled, but the main conclusion that calprotectin has a good diagnostic precision, especially in adults is well documented.

2.3.3 Calprotectin and differentiating between UC and CD

The test seems not useful for differentiating between the two diseases (Canani *et al.*, 2006; Silberer *et al.*, 2005; Tibble *et al.*, 2002; von Roon *et al.*, 2007). When comparing the sensitivity and specificity of calprotectin with other serological tests as CRP, ESR, ANCA or ASCA, calprotectin turn out as the best test in level with clinical scores (Gisbert *et al.*, 2009;Tibble *et al.*, 2002). Tibble et al included 602 patients where 263 had organic intestinal disease and 339 had nonorganic disease (Tibble *et al.*, 2002). Interestingly they found that both fecal calprotectin level and the Rome I criteria were significantly better screening discriminates of patients with organic or nonorganic intestinal disease (Odds ratio (OR), 27.8, positive predicative value (PPV), 0.76, negative predicative value (NPV), 0.89 and 13.3, 0.86, 0.69) than some other commonly used laboratory parameters, such as CRP (OR, 4.2, PPV, 0.67, NPV, 0.68) and ESR (OR, 3.2, PPV, 0.62, NPV, 0.69) (Tibble *et al.*, 2002). Other studies have listed comparable values (Canani *et al.*, 2006; Fagerberg *et al.*, 2005; Tibble *et al.*, 2000a). Sensitivity of calprotectin ranged from 92-95% and specificity ranged from 93-98%, while sensitivity of CRP ranged from 36-41% and specificity from 77-100%. For ESR the values ranged from 41-59% and specificity from 77-100%. For ASCA/PANCA, the sensitivity was 77% and specificity was 88% (Canani *et al.*, 2006).

2.3.4 Calprotectin and relapse in IBD

Tibbel et al have addressed whether calprotectin predict relapse in IBD (Tibble *et al.*, 2000b). They observed that at 50 microgram/gram, the sensitivity and specificity of calprotectin for predicting relapse in all patients with IBD were 90% and 83%, respectively. In their study calprotectin levels of 50 microgram/gram or more predicted a 13-fold increased risk for relapse. They did not find CRP or ESR to be useful in predicting relapse of IBD (Tibble *et al.*, 2000b). Other studies have confirmed the results of Tibbel et al (Costa *et al.*, 2005; D'Inca *et al.*, 2008).

2.3.5 Calprotectin and correlation with disease activity in IBD

Several studies have investigated and found a correlation between calprotectin and the severity of IBD evaluated with clinical, endoscopic and histologic parameters (Berni *et al.*, 2004; Langhorst *et al.*, 2005; Tibble *et al.*, 2000a; Tibble and Bjarnason, 2001). However, calprotectin seems to be better correlated with disease activity in UC than in CD (Costa *et al.*, 2003; D'Inca *et al.*, 2007). Though, it is important to have in mind that CDAI score is mostly based on clinical information and not sensitive concerning subclinical inflammation.

2.3.6 Calprotectin as a marker of treatment response in IBD

It is plausible that calprotectin decreases if a treated IBD patient achieves remission, but so far few studies have confirmed this hypothesis. In a small recent study 38 IBD patients were included and calprotectin was measured before and after treatment with topical/or systemic 5-ASA or prednisolon or immunosuppressiva (Wagner *et al.*, 2008). Using calprotectin values below 95th percentile of the normal range as a negative predictor of active disease after 8 week of treatment, they revealed a negative predicative value of 100%. However, using an elevated level of calprotectin as a positive predictor to detect ongoing active disease or treatment failure after 8 week of treatment, they calculated a positive predicative value of 38% in UC and only of 14% in CD (Wagner *et al.*, 2008). Comparable results were demonstrated in another study, including 57 children with IBD treated with prednisolon (Kolho *et al.*, 2006). In their series, the positive predicative value of fecal calprotectin for active IBD judged by colonoscopy was 0.7. They observed that calprotectin levels declined in line with the clinical improvement but seldom fell within the normal range. The authors suggested that this may be caused of an ongoing inflammation in a clinically silent disease

(Kolho *et al.,* 2006). An interesting study by Røseth et al included 45 IBD patients with normal calprotectin levels after treatment and demonstrated that in 44 of the 45 patients the appearance of both the colon and the terminal ileum was completely normal endoscopically (Roseth *et al.,* 2004). Sensitive markers of mucosal healing in IBD are urgently needed and this small study indicates that calprotectin could be such a marker in IBD patients. Future properly powered studies are needed to evaluate calprotectin as a possible marker of successful treatment in IBD.

2.3.7 Summary

As concluded in the systematic review by von Rheenen et al, high concentration of calprotectin in feces is a strong argument to carry out a colonoscopy in order to rule out the presence of inflammatory bowel disease or other organic pathologies. Parallelism between fecal calprotectin levels and inflammatory bowel disease activity has been confirmed, although this fecal marker appears to better reflect the disease activity in UC than in CD. Further, increased calprotectin levels are found to predict increased risk for relapse in IBD. However, the test seems not useful for differentiating between the two diseases. Finally, calprotectin have a good diagnostic precision for separating IBD from non-IBD diagnosis overall, better than classically ESR, CRP, ANCA or ASCA.

3. Histological parameters as predictors of disease severity or treatment response in IBD

To our knowledge there are not many studies done addressing histological parameters as predictors of disease severity or treatment outcome in IBD. After several search in pubmed.com we managed to find only one study published in 1993 (Schumacher, 1993). Schumacher investigated the possibilities of differentiating between inflammatory bowel disease (IBD) and infectious colitis on clinical, microbiological, laboratory and histological grounds, a prospective study of 105 patients with a first attack of colitis was undertaken (Schumacher, 1993). The strongest histological predictor of IBD in this study was basal plasmocytosis, followed by more than two vertical crypt branches/MPF, crypt distortion, villous mucosa, mucosal atrophy, epithelioid granulomas and Paneth cell metaplasia. These signs were rarely or never found among patients with infectious colitis. Their frequency increased with the interval between the initial symptoms and the first biopsy. Lately, researchers have been focusing on other biomarkers in serum, faeces or mucosa in IBD patients searching for possible predictors of both disease activity and treatment response and compared these biomarkers with both histology and endoscopy in IBD patients.

4. Mucosal inflammatory processes: The main source of biomarkers in IBD

4.1 Introduction

The biological tissue factors playing a role in the pro-inflammatory and anti-inflammatory process in IBD have been revealed by the omics technology and described in several overviews (Kaser *et al.,* 2010;Neuman, 2007;Torres and Rios, 2008): microarray and quantitative real-time polymerase chain reaction (RT-PCR) analyses describe the gene expression of IBD-related proteins, the proteomics describe the translation of proteins including small oligopeptides, whereas the metabolomics describe all the metabolic endproducts of gene expressions. This gives a unique option for molecular fingerprinting. In general, these tissue factors are linked to various immunological pathways belonging to the innate, adaptive and regulatory immune response including molecules such as cytokines, chemokines, adhesion molecules and other markers of activation with corresponding cellular and soluble receptors; immune cells and non-immune cells. Finally, a relatively new field in IBD, the metabolic fingerprints obtained from metabolomics studies (for review, see (Roda *et al.*, 2010; Scaldaferri *et al.*, 2010). So far there are few reports describing prognostic and predictive bioamarkers. In the following we will describe the candidate biomarkers predicting either clinical outcomes and/or response to therapy. Moreover, as there are very few documented biomarkers we will also add some molecules central in the inflammatory process in IBD that is of great interest in the future biomarker fingerprinting based on the new approaches in high technological omics.

4.2 Proinflammatory cytokines

4.2.1 TNF-α

TNF-α is a cytokine well established inflammatory mediator of CD whereas contradictory reports exist in UC (Kaser *et al.*, 2010; Neuman, 2007;Torres and Rios, 2008). Some reports have found positive correlations with the degree of disease activity in UC (Akazawa *et al.*, 2002;Olsen *et al.*, 2007) and CD (Olsen *et al.*, 2007) but not in all for CD (Akazawa *et al.*, 2002) and UC (Dionne *et al.*, 1997).
As far as we know no studies do exist on mucosal expressions of TNF-α and the prediction of the clinical course, whereas there are only few reports on the predictive value of mucosal TNF-α concentrations and the response to therapy. Pretreatment mucosal TNF-α concentrations were negatively correlated to response to Infliximab in CD (Schmidt *et al.*, 2007) and in UC (Olsen *et al.*, 2007). These findings disagree with another report where low expression of TNF-α predicted a poor response to therapy in CD (Arsenescu *et al.*, 2008). Increased levels of TNF-α were also observed in corticosteroid non-responders compared with responders to corticosteroid treatment in UC (Ishiguro, 1999), but not confirmed in another study (Raddatz *et al.*, 2005). Finally, in a preliminary report, normalization of mucosal TNF-α seemed to predict a longstanding remission after stop of anti-TNF therapy both in UC (Olsen T *et al.*, 2011a). Finally, based on microarray technology in UC patients treated with nfliximab expression of TNF-receptor (SF11B), the receptor for the proinflammatory cytokine 13 (IL-13-R) and the anti-inflammatory cytokine IL-11 predicted the clinical response

4.2.2 IFN-γ, IL-1, IL-12

TNF-α exerts its proinflammatory effect through cytokines such as INF-γ, IL-1β and IL-6 (Neuman, 2007). INF-γ is a mediator of inflammation in CD (Strober *et al.*, 2010), whereas contradictory reports exist for UC (Kobayashi *et al.*, 2008; Olsen *et al.*, 2007). Finally, in one report increased levels of INF-γ in intestinal T lymphocyte cultures were observed in relapsing perianal fistulising disease in CD after treatment with infliximab (Agnholt *et al.*, 2003).
IL-1β was increased in CD and UC in one report (Dionne *et al.*, 1998), and IL-1-receptor/IL-1β ratio is negatively associated to the IBD activity (Dionne *et al.*, 1998). IL-12 is a proinflammatory cytokine known for gating (in synergy with IL-18) in a Th1 direction/stimulating the IFN-γ synthesis in naïve T cells and is up-regulated in IBD (Neuman, 2007). IL-12 in addition to INF-γ and IL-6 is more increased in inflamed than in not inflamed mucosa (Leon *et al.*, 2009). However, neither of these cytokines has been studied as potential biomarkers

4.2.3 IL-6

IL-6 is a pleiotropic cytokine with regulatory effects on the inflammation. The cytokine plays an important role in the initial activation of immune response and in combination with the transforming growth factor (TGF-β), plays a pivotal role in TH17 polarization. Increased levels of the cytokine and its soluble receptor are increased in active CD and in UC (for review, see (Atreya and Neurath, 2005)), but their roles as biomarker are so unknown.

4.2.4 IL-17/Il-23

The first reports of increased density of IL-17 cells in the inflamed mucosa of IBD came in 2003 (Fujino *et al.*, 2003) and was confirmed by later studies (Kobayashi *et al.*, 2008; Olsen T *et al.*, 2011b). Both IL-17 and IL-23 are correlated to the severity of UC (Olsen T *et al.*, 2011b) and are positive correlated to the response to infliximab (Olsen T *et al.*, 2010). Homozygous carriers of IBD risk-increasing IL-23 receptor variants are more likely to respond to infliximab (Jurgens *et al.*, 2010).

4.3 Antiinflammatory cytokines

4.3.1 Transforming growth factor-β

Transforming growth factor-β1 (TGF-β1) is a potent regulatory cytokine, and has in the absence of IL-6, an antiinflammatory effect. Increased levels of TGF-β1 are found both in CD and UC (Lawrance *et al.*, 2001; Olsen T *et al.*, 2011b), which are correlated with the severity of disease in CD but not in UC (Olsen T *et al.*, 2011b).

4.3.2 IL-10

IL-10 has anti-inflammatory effects on proinflammatory cytokines (IL-1, IL-6, TNF-α) and its mucosal levels were found increased both in CD and UC (Akagi *et al.*, 2000; Olsen *et al.*, 2007) (for review see(Kaser *et al.*, 2010)) except for a single study(Nielsen *et al.*, 1996). Of interest, mucosal levels of IL-10 and IL-4 in UC did not correlate with the treatment effects of infliximab (Olsen *et al.*, 2009) and were not found reduced after infliximab treatment (Agnholt *et al.*, 2003).

4.3.3 IL-11

IL-11 mediates anti-inflammatory effects by downregulation of LPS-induced NFkB activation preceding transcription of inflammatory genes. In the mucosal gene signature study of Arijs et al (Arijs *et al.*, 2009) (39) IL-11 was one of several expressed genes separating responders from non-responders on infliximab treatment.

4.4 Molecules of activation

4.4.1 Adhesion molecules and chemokines

4.4.1.1 The adhesion molecules play an important role in mediating intestinal injury by T cells in IBD

The endothelium plays a key role in the pathogenesis of IBD acting as "gatekeeper" regulating the leukocyte trafficking through cell adhesion molecules and chemokine secretion. Integrins, selectins and immunoglobulins are receptors on leukocytes, endothelium, and platelets with their respective ligands which are up-regulated by proinflammatory cytokines through a NF-κB dependent mechanism. Integrin α4β7 expressed on lymphocytes and its specific ligand mucosal vascular addressin on the endothelial cells play a pivotal role in the recruitment of leucocytes from blood to the inflamed tissue. An increased expressions of several adhesion molecules such as e-selectin, intracellular adhesion molecule-1 and 2 (ICAM-1, ICAM 2) and vascular cell adhesion molecule (VCAM) have been found in IBD (for review see (Danese *et al.*, 2005). Although the leukocyte recruitment by adhesion molecules plays a role in the initiation and progression of the disease, there is little documentation of their roles as biomarkers. The gene expression of ICAM-1 is elevated in UC but was not correlated with response to steroids (Raddatz *et al.*, 2004). In the same study low expression of the glucocorticoid receptor was correlated to non-response. Of interest, in the study of Nicolaus et al (Nikolaus *et al.*, 2000) relapsers after induction therapy with infliximab in CD were characterized by an increase in the TNF-α secretion capacity and increased mucosal nuclear NF-κB p65 before recurrence of clinical symptoms. Chemokines and their corresponding receptors are responsible for the chemotaxis and the adhesion and directional homing of immune and inflammatory cells from blood to tissue. The exact immunopathogenic role of chemokines in IBD is not clearly understood. However, increased tissue expressions of these molecules in IBD reflect increased trafficking and lymphocytes recirculation and neo-lympho organogenesis in the intestinal mucosa mediating not only inflammatory process but also repair mechanisms (for review see (Zimmerman *et al.*, 2008)).

4.4.2 Markers of tissue injury

Among the effector mechanisms activated during intestinal inflammation are the key mediators such as inducible nitric oxide synthase (INOS), the apoptosis-related Granzyme B (GZNB), and the system of extracellular matrix degradation mediated by metalloproteinases (MMP). The pathophysiological role of nitric oxide in IBD is to some extent controversial. Increased INOS activity has been shown especially in UC (Palatka *et al.*, 2005) and predicted the progression in IBD (Menchen *et al.*, 2004). Some of MMPs are proinflammatory and found dysregulated in IBD (MMP-1,-3,-9, -12, -13) (Ravi *et al.*, 2007; von *et al.*, 2000). The tissue inhibitor of MMPs (TIMP) has reported to correlate both, positively (macrophage TIMP-1) and negatively (epithelial TIMP-3) to the disease activity in CD, whereas MMPs and TIMPs were decreased after treatment of the disease (Makitalo *et al.*, 2009). In one report infliximab reduced a genotype-associated matrix protective phenotype (Meijer *et al.*, 2007).

4.4.3 Genomics

There is increasing number of IBD suspectibility loci/genes discovered. There is beyond the goal of this review of mucosal biomarkers to describe the genomics in IBD. In short, the most powerful tool is the use of genome-wide association (GWA) scanning in genotyping. In 2011, 71 and 47 suspectibility loci/genes have been discovered in CD and UD, respectively, including 28 in common comprising the total number of 99 loci involved. (Anderson *et al.*, 2011;Franke *et al.*, 2010). This genetic polymorphism linked to the innate immunity, autophagy, defective barrier, IL-10 signalling and adaptive immunity. Of these suspectibility loci/genes some have also been candidate biomarkers. Polymorphisms in apoptopic genes (Fas/LFas system and caspace-9 influence the response of infliximab in luminal and fistulising Crohn's disease (Hlavaty *et al.*, 2005). Using GWA technology a loci (21q22,212IBRWDI) remained significant for responsiveness to anti TNF therapy in children (Franke *et al.*, 2010). There are now several IBD studies worldwide using the GWA technology and functional genomics. Hopefully, these genome analyses together with gene expression analyses can define new subtypes of clinical outcomes and response to various treatment regimes.

4.4.4 Proteomics

Proteomics identifies biomarkers at protein expression levels in tissue and opens for protein dynamic mapping of proteins in the inflammatory pathways and their metabolic end products. So far, no mucosal proteomics have been reported in IBD, whereas 4 biomarkers of acute phase inflammation have been found in serum from patients with IBD (Meuwis *et al.*, 2008a) and the chemokine platelet aggregation factor 4 (PF4) in serum predicted the response to infliximab in CD (Meuwis *et al.*, 2008b). Of special interest is the fingerprinting of oxidative stress in inflammation and modification of proteins and thereby new potential biomarkers. So far, we are waiting for prospective studies relating fingerprints in mucosa to severity of disease and predictors to treatment.

4.4.5 Metabolomics

Metalobomics is the study of chemical fingerprints of all metabolites in the biological organism and represents the end product of the gene transcriptions. By the use of nuclear magnetic resonance (NMR) spectroscopy and mass spectrometry (MS) simultaneously assessment of numerous of metabolites corresponding to the "metabolome" and its end-points of metabolic products may be done. Thus, in UC different metabolic profiles have been observed in biopsies when compared to controls (Bjerrum *et al.*, 2010). In CD, pathways with differentiating metabolites included those involved in the metabolism and or synthesis of amino acids, fatty acids, bile acids and arachidonic acid, several metabolites were positively or negatively correlated to the disease phenotype (Jansson *et al.*, 2009). Finally, in fecal extracts low levels of butyrate and acetate and amino acids have been observed in IBD compared to the controls (Marchesi *et al.*, 2007). This opens for new insight of the etiopathogenesis of the disease. However, so far we do not know how this technology can contribute to the discovery of new biomarkers.

5. Concluding remarks

There are so far very few documentations of mucosal (by biopsy) or body fluid (non-invasive) biomarkers predicting long-term clinical outcome or response to treatment. The most promising candidate predictors are TNF-α but no validation data exists. In general, there is a need for prospective studies with a broad fingerprinting assay from mucosa as well as from body fluids. From a theoretical point of view, mediators of inflammation and their metabolites correlating with severity of disease are the candidates of greatest interest. After documentation of a candidate biomarker, there is a need of both a validation and adjustments of practical use for the clinicians. Therefore, biomarkers of IBD are still in the start of defining candidates of interest.

6. References

(2010) Valid concerns. *Nature*, 463, 401-402.

Agnholt, J., Dahlerup, J. F., Buntzen, S., Tottrup, A., Nielsen, S. L., Lundorf, E. (2003) Response, relapse and mucosal immune regulation after infliximab treatment in fistulating Crohn's disease. *Aliment.Pharmacol.Ther.*, 17, 703-710.

Aisenberg, J., Legnani, P. E., Nilubol, N., Cobrin, G. M., Ellozy, S. H., Hegazi, R. A., Yager, J., Bodian, C., Gorfine, S. R., Bauer, J. J., Plevy, S. E., Sachar, D. B. (2004) Are pANCA, ASCA, or cytokine gene polymorphisms associated with pouchitis? Long-term follow-up in 102 ulcerative colitis patients. *Am.J.Gastroenterol.*, 99, 432-441.

Akagi, S., Hiyama, E., Imamura, Y., Takesue, Y., Matsuura, Y., Yokoyama, T. (2000) Interleukin-10 expression in intestine of Crohn disease. *Int.J.Mol.Med.*, 5, 389-395.

Akazawa, A., Sakaida, I., Higaki, S., Kubo, Y., Uchida, K., Okita, K. (2002) Increased expression of tumor necrosis factor-alpha messenger RNA in the intestinal mucosa of inflammatory bowel disease, particularly in patients with disease in the inactive phase. *J.Gastroenterol.*, 37, 345-353.

Anderson, C. A., Boucher, G., Lees, C. W., Franke, A., D'Amato, M., Taylor, K. D., Lee, J. C., Goyette, P., Imielinski, M., Latiano, A., Lagace, C., Scott, R., Amininejad, L., Bumpstead, S., Baidoo, L., Baldassano, R. N., Barclay, M., Bayless, T. M., Brand, S., Buning, C., Colombel, J. F., Denson, L. A., De, V. M., Dubinsky, M., Edwards, C., Ellinghaus, D., Fehrmann, R. S., Floyd, J. A., Florin, T., Franchimont, D., Franke, L., Georges, M., Glas, J., Glazer, N. L., Guthery, S. L., Haritunians, T., Hayward, N. K., Hugot, J. P., Jobin, G., Laukens, D., Lawrance, I., Lemann, M., Levine, A., Libioulle, C., Louis, E., McGovern, D. P., Milla, M., Montgomery, G. W., Morley, K. I., Mowat, C., Ng, A., Newman, W., Ophoff, R. A., Papi, L., Palmieri, O., Peyrin-Biroulet, L., Panes, J., Phillips, A., Prescott, N. J., Proctor, D. D., Roberts, R., Russell, R., Rutgeerts, P., Sanderson, J., Sans, M., Schumm, P., Seibold, F., Sharma, Y., Simms, L. A., Seielstad, M., Steinhart, A. H., Targan, S. R., van den Berg, L. H., Vatn, M., Verspaget, H., Walters, T., Wijmenga, C., Wilson, D. C., Westra, H. J., Xavier, R. J., Zhao, Z. Z., Ponsioen, C. Y., Andersen, V., Torkvist, L., Gazouli, M., Anagnou, N. P., Karlsen, T. H., Kupcinskas, L., Sventoraityte, J., Mansfield, J. C., Kugathasan, S., Silverberg, M. S., Halfvarson, J., Rotter, J. I., Mathew, C. G., Griffiths, A. M., Gearry, R., Ahmad, T., Brant, S. R., Chamaillard, M., Satsangi, J., Cho, J. H., Schreiber, S., Daly, M. J., Barrett, J. C., Parkes, M., Annese, V., Hakonarson, H., Radford-Smith, G., Duerr, R. H., Vermeire, S., Weersma, R. K., Rioux, J. D. (2011) Meta-analysis identifies 29 additional ulcerative colitis risk loci, increasing the number of confirmed associations to 47. *Nat.Genet.*, 43, 246-252.

Arijs, I., Li, K., Toedter, G., Quintens, R., Van, L. L., van, S. K., Leemans, P., De, H. G., Lemaire, K., Ferrante, M., Schnitzler, F., Thorrez, L., Ma, K., Song, X. Y., Marano, C., Van, A. G., Vermeire, S., Geboes, K., Schuit, F., Baribaud, F., Rutgeerts, P. (2009) Mucosal gene signatures to predict response to infliximab in patients with ulcerative colitis. *Gut*, 58, 1612-1619.

Arsenescu, R., Bruno, M. E., Rogier, E. W., Stefka, A. T., McMahan, A. E., Wright, T. B., Nasser, M. S., de Villiers, W. J., Kaetzel, C. S. (2008) Signature biomarkers in Crohn's disease: toward a molecular classification. *Mucosal.Immunol.*, 1, 399-411.

Atreya, R., Neurath, M. F. (2005) Involvement of IL-6 in the pathogenesis of inflammatory bowel disease and colon cancer. *Clin.Rev.Allergy Immunol.*, 28, 187-196.

Berni, C. R., Rapacciuolo, L., Romano, M. T., Tanturri de, H. L., Terrin, G., Manguso, F., Cirillo, P., Paparo, F., Troncone, R. (2004) Diagnostic value of faecal calprotectin in paediatric gastroenterology clinical practice. *Dig.Liver Dis.*, 36, 467-470.

Bjerrum, J. T., Nielsen, O. H., Hao, F., Tang, H., Nicholson, J. K., Wang, Y., Olsen, J. (2010) Metabonomics in ulcerative colitis: diagnostics, biomarker identification, and insight into the pathophysiology. *J.Proteome.Res.*, 9, 954-962.

Calkins, B. M. (1989) A meta-analysis of the role of smoking in inflammatory bowel disease. *Dig.Dis.Sci.*, 34, 1841-1854.

Canani, R. B., de Horatio, L. T., Terrin, G., Romano, M. T., Miele, E., Staiano, A., Rapacciuolo, L., Polito, G., Bisesti, V., Manguso, F., Vallone, G., Sodano, A., Troncone, R. (2006) Combined use of noninvasive tests is useful in the initial diagnostic approach to a child with suspected inflammatory bowel disease. *J.Pediatr.Gastroenterol.Nutr.*, 42, 9-15.

Cario, E. (2010) Toll-like receptors in inflammatory bowel diseases: a decade later. *Inflamm.Bowel.Dis.*, 16, 1583-1597.

Carlson, C. S., Aldred, S. F., Lee, P. K., Tracy, R. P., Schwartz, S. M., Rieder, M., Liu, K., Williams, O. D., Iribarren, C., Lewis, E. C., Fornage, M., Boerwinkle, E., Gross, M., Jaquish, C., Nickerson, D. A., Myers, R. M., Siscovick, D. S., Reiner, A. P. (2005) Polymorphisms within the C-reactive protein (CRP) promoter region are associated with plasma CRP levels. *Am.J.Hum.Genet.*, 77, 64-77.

Carroccio, A., Iacono, G., Cottone, M., Di, P. L., Cartabellotta, F., Cavataio, F., Scalici, C., Montalto, G., Di, F. G., Rini, G., Notarbartolo, A., Averna, M. R. (2003) Diagnostic accuracy of fecal calprotectin assay in distinguishing organic causes of chronic diarrhea from irritable bowel syndrome: a prospective study in adults and children. *Clin.Chem.*, 49, 861-867.

Chouhan, S., Gahlot, S., Pokharna, R. K., Mathur, K. C., Saini, K., Pal, M. (2006) Severity and extent of ulcerative colitis: role of C-reactive protein. *Indian J.Gastroenterol.*, 25, 46-47.

Colburn, W. A. (2000) Optimizing the use of biomarkers, surrogate endpoints, and clinical endpoints for more efficient drug development. *J.Clin.Pharmacol.*, 40, 1419-1427.

Colombel, J. F., Solem, C. A., Sandborn, W. J., Booya, F., Loftus, E. V., Jr., Harmsen, W. S., Zinsmeister, A. R., Bodily, K. D., Fletcher, J. G. (2006) Quantitative measurement and visual assessment of ileal Crohn's disease activity by computed tomography enterography: correlation with endoscopic severity and C reactive protein. *Gut*, 55, 1561-1567.

Costa, F., Mumolo, M. G., Bellini, M., Romano, M. R., Ceccarelli, L., Arpe, P., Sterpi, C., Marchi, S., Maltinti, G. (2003) Role of faecal calprotectin as non-invasive marker of intestinal inflammation. *Dig.Liver Dis.*, 35, 642-647.

Costa, F., Mumolo, M. G., Ceccarelli, L., Bellini, M., Romano, M. R., Sterpi, C., Ricchiuti, A., Marchi, S., Bottai, M. (2005) Calprotectin is a stronger predictive marker of relapse in ulcerative colitis than in Crohn's disease. *Gut*, 54, 364-368.

D'Inca, R., Dal, P. E., Di, L., V, Benazzato, L., Martinato, M., Lamboglia, F., Oliva, L., Sturniolo, G. C. (2008) Can calprotectin predict relapse risk in inflammatory bowel disease? *Am.J.Gastroenterol.*, 103, 2007-2014.

D'Inca, R., Dal, P. E., Di, L., V, Ferronato, A., Fries, W., Vettorato, M. G., Martines, D., Sturniolo, G. C. (2007) Calprotectin and lactoferrin in the assessment of intestinal inflammation and organic disease. *Int.J.Colorectal Dis.*, 22, 429-437.

Danese, S., Semeraro, S., Marini, M., Roberto, I., Armuzzi, A., Papa, A., Gasbarrini, A. (2005) Adhesion molecules in inflammatory bowel disease: therapeutic implications for gut inflammation. *Dig.Liver Dis.*, 37, 811-818.

Dionne, S., D'Agata, I. D., Hiscott, J., Vanounou, T., Seidman, E. G. (1998) Colonic explant production of IL-1and its receptor antagonist is imbalanced in inflammatory bowel disease (IBD). *Clin.Exp.Immunol.*, 112, 435-442.

Dionne, S., Hiscott, J., D'Agata, I., Duhaime, A., Seidman, E. G. (1997) Quantitative PCR analysis of TNF-alpha and IL-1 beta mRNA levels in pediatric IBD mucosal biopsies. *Dig.Dis.Sci.*, 42, 1557-1566.

Eaden, J. A., Abrams, K. R., Mayberry, J. F. (2001) The risk of colorectal cancer in ulcerative colitis: a meta-analysis. *Gut*, 48, 526-535.

Fagerberg, U. L., Loof, L., Myrdal, U., Hansson, L. O., Finkel, Y. (2005) Colorectal inflammation is well predicted by fecal calprotectin in children with gastrointestinal symptoms. *J.Pediatr.Gastroenterol.Nutr.*, 40, 450-455.

Fantuzzi, G. (2005) Adipose tissue, adipokines, and inflammation. *J.Allergy Clin.Immunol.*, 115, 911-919.

Ferrante, M., Vermeire, S., Katsanos, K. H., Noman, M., Van, A. G., Schnitzler, F., Arijs, I., De, H. G., Hoffman, I., Geboes, J. K., Rutgeerts, P. (2007) Predictors of early response to infliximab in patients with ulcerative colitis. *Inflamm.Bowel.Dis.*, 13, 123-128.

Fleshner, P. R., Vasiliauskas, E. A., Kam, L. Y., Fleshner, N. E., Gaiennie, J., breu-Martin, M. T., Targan, S. R. (2001) High level perinuclear antineutrophil cytoplasmic antibody (pANCA) in ulcerative colitis patients before colectomy predicts the development of chronic pouchitis after ileal pouch-anal anastomosis. *Gut*, 49, 671-677.

Franke, A., McGovern, D. P., Barrett, J. C., Wang, K., Radford-Smith, G. L., Ahmad, T., Lees, C. W., Balschun, T., Lee, J., Roberts, R., Anderson, C. A., Bis, J. C., Bumpstead, S., Ellinghaus, D., Festen, E. M., Georges, M., Green, T., Haritunians, T., Jostins, L., Latiano, A., Mathew, C. G., Montgomery, G. W., Prescott, N. J., Raychaudhuri, S., Rotter, J. I., Schumm, P., Sharma, Y., Simms, L. A., Taylor, K. D., Whiteman, D., Wijmenga, C., Baldassano, R. N., Barclay, M., Bayless, T. M., Brand, S., Buning, C., Cohen, A., Colombel, J. F., Cottone, M., Stronati, L., Denson, T., De, V. M., D'Inca, R., Dubinsky, M., Edwards, C., Florin, T., Franchimont, D., Gearry, R., Glas, J., Van, G. A., Guthery, S. L., Halfvarson, J., Verspaget, H. W., Hugot, J. P., Karban, A., Laukens, D., Lawrance, I., Lemann, M., Levine, A., Libioulle, C., Louis, E., Mowat, C., Newman, W., Panes, J., Phillips, A., Proctor, D. D., Regueiro, M., Russell, R., Rutgeerts, P., Sanderson, J., Sans, M., Seibold, F., Steinhart, A. H., Stokkers, P. C., Torkvist, L., Kullak-Ublick, G., Wilson, D., Walters, T., Targan, S. R., Brant, S. R., Rioux, J. D., D'Amato, M., Weersma, R. K., Kugathasan, S., Griffiths, A. M., Mansfield, J. C., Vermeire, S., Duerr, R. H., Silverberg, M. S., Satsangi, J., Schreiber, S., Cho, J. H., Annese, V., Hakonarson, H., Daly, M. J., Parkes, M. (2010) Genome-wide meta-analysis increases to 71 the number of confirmed Crohn's disease susceptibility loci. *Nat.Genet.*, 42, 1118-1125.

Fujino, S., Andoh, A., Bamba, S., Ogawa, A., Hata, K., Araki, Y., Bamba, T., Fujiyama, Y. (2003) Increased expression of interleukin 17 in inflammatory bowel disease. *Gut*, 52, 65-70.

Gisbert, J. P., McNicholl, A. G., Gomollon, F. (2009) Questions and answers on the role of fecal lactoferrin as a biological marker in inflammatory bowel disease. *Inflamm.Bowel.Dis.*, 15, 1746-1754.

Greenfield, J. R., Samaras, K., Jenkins, A. B., Kelly, P. J., Spector, T. D., Gallimore, J. R., Pepys, M. B., Campbell, L. V. (2004) Obesity is an important determinant of baseline serum C-reactive protein concentration in monozygotic twins, independent of genetic influences. *Circulation*, 109, 3022-3028.

Henriksen, M., Jahnsen, J., Lygren, I., Stray, N., Sauar, J., Vatn, M. H., Moum, B. (2008) C-reactive protein: a predictive factor and marker of inflammation in inflammatory bowel disease. Results from a prospective population-based study. *Gut*, 57, 1518-1523.

Hlavaty, T., Pierik, M., Henckaerts, L., Ferrante, M., Joossens, S., Van, S. N., Noman, M., Rutgeerts, P., Vermeire, S. (2005) Polymorphisms in apoptosis genes predict response to infliximab therapy in luminal and fistulizing Crohn's disease. *Aliment.Pharmacol.Ther.*, 22, 613-626.

Hoie, O., Wolters, F., Riis, L., Aamodt, G., Solberg, C., Bernklev, T., Odes, S., Mouzas, I. A., Beltrami, M., Langholz, E., Stockbrugger, R., Vatn, M., Moum, B. (2007) Ulcerative colitis: patient characteristics may predict 10-yr disease recurrence in a European-wide population-based cohort. *Am.J.Gastroenterol.*, 102, 1692-1701.

Isakson, P., Hammarstedt, A., Gustafson, B., Smith, U. (2009) Impaired Preadipocyte differentiation in human abdominal obesity: role of Wnt, tumor necrosis factor-alpha, and inflammation. *Diabetes*, 58, 1550-1557.

Ishiguro, Y. (1999) Mucosal proinflammatory cytokine production correlates with endoscopic activity of ulcerative colitis. *J.Gastroenterol.*, 34, 66-74.

Jansson, J., Willing, B., Lucio, M., Fekete, A., Dicksved, J., Halfvarson, J., Tysk, C., Schmitt-Kopplin, P. (2009) Metabolomics reveals metabolic biomarkers of Crohn's disease. *PLoS.One.*, 4, e6386.

Joossens, S., Reinisch, W., Vermeire, S., Sendid, B., Poulain, D., Peeters, M., Geboes, K., Bossuyt, X., Vandewalle, P., Oberhuber, G., Vogelsang, H., Rutgeerts, P., Colombel, J. F. (2002) The value of serologic markers in indeterminate colitis: a prospective follow-up study. *Gastroenterology*, 122, 1242-1247.

Jurgens, M., Laubender, R. P., Hartl, F., Weidinger, M., Seiderer, J., Wagner, J., Wetzke, M., Beigel, F., Pfennig, S., Stallhofer, J., Schnitzler, F., Tillack, C., Lohse, P., Goke, B., Glas, J., Ochsenkuhn, T., Brand, S. (2010) Disease activity, ANCA, and IL23R genotype status determine early response to infliximab in patients with ulcerative colitis. *Am.J.Gastroenterol.*, 105, 1811-1819.

Kaser, A., Zeissig, S., Blumberg, R. S. (2010) Inflammatory bowel disease. *Annu.Rev.Immunol.*, 28, 573-621.

Kobayashi, T., Okamoto, S., Hisamatsu, T., Kamada, N., Chinen, H., Saito, R., Kitazume, M. T., Nakazawa, A., Sugita, A., Koganei, K., Isobe, K. I., Hibi, T. (2008) IL-23 differentially regulates the Th1/Th17 balance in ulcerative colitis and Crohn's disease. *Gut*.

Kolho, K. L., Raivio, T., Lindahl, H., Savilahti, E. (2006) Fecal calprotectin remains high during glucocorticoid therapy in children with inflammatory bowel disease. *Scand.J.Gastroenterol.*, 41, 720-725.

Langhorst, J., Elsenbruch, S., Mueller, T., Rueffer, A., Spahn, G., Michalsen, A., Dobos, G. J. (2005) Comparison of 4 neutrophil-derived proteins in feces as indicators of disease activity in ulcerative colitis. *Inflamm.Bowel.Dis.*, 11, 1085-1091.

Lawrance, I. C., Maxwell, L., Doe, W. (2001) Inflammation location, but not type, determines the increase in TGF-beta1 and IGF-1 expression and collagen deposition in IBD intestine. *Inflamm.Bowel.Dis.*, 7, 16-26.

Leon, A. J., Gomez, E., Garrote, J. A., Bernardo, D., Barrera, A., Marcos, J. L., Fernandez-Salazar, L., Velayos, B., Blanco-Quiros, A., Arranz, E. (2009) High levels of proinflammatory cytokines, but not markers of tissue injury, in unaffected intestinal areas from patients with IBD. *Mediators.Inflamm.*, 2009, 580450.

Lewis, J. D. (2011) The utility of biomarkers in the diagnosis and therapy of inflammatory bowel disease. *Gastroenterology*, 140, 1817-1826.

Lundberg, J. O., Hellstrom, P. M., Fagerhol, M. K., Weitzberg, E., Roseth, A. G. (2005) Technology insight: calprotectin, lactoferrin and nitric oxide as novel markers of inflammatory bowel disease. *Nat.Clin.Pract.Gastroenterol.Hepatol.*, 2, 96-102.

Macdonald, J. K., McDonald, J. W. (2007) Natalizumab for induction of remission in Crohn's disease. *Cochrane.Database.Syst.Rev.*, CD006097.

Makitalo, L., Sipponen, T., Karkkainen, P., Kolho, K. L., Saarialho-Kere, U. (2009) Changes in matrix metalloproteinase (MMP) and tissue inhibitors of metalloproteinases (TIMP) expression profile in Crohn's disease after immunosuppressive treatment correlate with histological score and calprotectin values. *Int.J.Colorectal Dis.*, 24, 1157-1167.

Marchesi, J. R., Holmes, E., Khan, F., Kochhar, S., Scanlan, P., Shanahan, F., Wilson, I. D., Wang, Y. (2007) Rapid and noninvasive metabonomic characterization of inflammatory bowel disease. *J.Proteome.Res.*, 6, 546-551.

Meijer, M. J., Mieremet-Ooms, M. A., van, D. W., van der Zon, A. M., Hanemaaijer, R., Verheijen, J. H., van Hogezand, R. A., Lamers, C. B., Verspaget, H. W. (2007) Effect of the anti-tumor necrosis factor-alpha antibody infliximab on the ex vivo mucosal matrix metalloproteinase-proteolytic phenotype in inflammatory bowel disease. *Inflamm.Bowel.Dis.*, 13, 200-210.

Menchen, L., Colon, A. L., Madrigal, J. L., Beltran, L., Botella, S., Lizasoain, I., Leza, J. C., Moro, M. A., Menchen, P., Cos, E., Lorenzo, P. (2004) Activity of inducible and neuronal nitric oxide synthases in colonic mucosa predicts progression of ulcerative colitis. *Am.J.Gastroenterol.*, 99, 1756-1764.

Mendoza, J. L., Abreu, M. T. (2009) Biological markers in inflammatory bowel disease: practical consideration for clinicians. *Gastroenterol.Clin.Biol.*, 33 Suppl 3, S158-S173.

Meuwis, M. A., Fillet, M., Chapelle, J. P., Malaise, M., Louis, E., Merville, M. P. (2008a) New biomarkers of Crohn's disease: serum biomarkers and development of diagnostic tools. *Expert.Rev.Mol.Diagn.*, 8, 327-337.

Meuwis, M. A., Fillet, M., Lutteri, L., Maree, R., Geurts, P., de, S. D., Malaise, M., Chapelle, J. P., Wehenkel, L., Belaiche, J., Merville, M. P., Louis, E. (2008b) Proteomics for prediction and characterization of response to infliximab in Crohn's disease: a pilot study. *Clin.Biochem.*, 41, 960-967.

Mow, W. S., Vasiliauskas, E. A., Lin, Y. C., Fleshner, P. R., Papadakis, K. A., Taylor, K. D., Landers, C. J., breu-Martin, M. T., Rotter, J. I., Yang, H., Targan, S. R. (2004)

Association of antibody responses to microbial antigens and complications of small bowel Crohn's disease. *Gastroenterology*, 126, 414-424.

Neuman, M. G. (2007) Immune dysfunction in inflammatory bowel disease. *Transl.Res.*, 149, 173-186.

Nielsen, O. H., Koppen, T., Rudiger, N., Horn, T., Eriksen, J., Kirman, I. (1996) Involvement of interleukin-4 and -10 in inflammatory bowel disease. *Dig.Dis.Sci.*, 41, 1786-1793.

Nikolaus, S., Raedler, A., Kuhbacker, T., Sfikas, N., Folsch, U. R., Schreiber, S. (2000) Mechanisms in failure of infliximab for Crohn's disease. *Lancet*, 356, 1475-1479.

Olsen T, Rismo R, Goll R, Cui G, Christiansen I, Florholmen J (2010) IL-17 gene expression in colorectal mucosa as a predictor of remission after induction therapy with infliximab in ulcerative colitis. In p. 1.

Olsen T, Rismo R, G. R., Cui G, Christiansen I, F. J. (2011a) Normalization of Mucosal TNF-alpha as a criterion when to stop treatment with anti TNF in UC patients? In p. S24.

Olsen T, R. R. e. d., Cui G, Goll R, Christiansen I, Husebekk A, Florholmen J (2011b) TH1 and TH17 interactions in untreated inflamed mucosa of inflammatory bowel disease. In Submitted Cytokine (ed).

Olsen, T., Cui, G., Goll, R., Husebekk, A., Florholmen, J. (2009) Infliximab therapy decreases the levels of TNF-alpha and IFN-gamma mRNA in colonic mucosa of ulcerative colitis. *Scand.J.Gastroenterol.*, 44, 727-735.

Olsen, T., Goll, R., Cui, G., Husebekk, A., Vonen, B., Birketvedt, G. S., Florholmen, J. (2007) Tissue levels of tumor necrosis factor-alpha correlates with grade of inflammation in untreated ulcerative colitis. *Scand.J.Gastroenterol.*, 42, 1312-1320.

Palatka, K., Serfozo, Z., Vereb, Z., Hargitay, Z., Lontay, B., Erdodi, F., Banfalvi, G., Nemes, Z., Udvardy, M., Altorjay, I. (2005) Changes in the expression and distribution of the inducible and endothelial nitric oxide synthase in mucosal biopsy specimens of inflammatory bowel disease. *Scand.J.Gastroenterol.*, 40, 670-680.

Pepys, M. B., Hirschfield, G. M. (2003) C-reactive protein: a critical update. *J.Clin.Invest*, 111, 1805-1812.

Prantera, C., Davoli, M., Lorenzetti, R., Pallone, F., Marcheggiano, A., Iannoni, C., Mariotti, S. (1988) Clinical and laboratory indicators of extent of ulcerative colitis. Serum C-reactive protein helps the most. *J.Clin.Gastroenterol.*, 10, 41-45.

Raddatz, D., Bockemuhl, M., Ramadori, G. (2005) Quantitative measurement of cytokine mRNA in inflammatory bowel disease: relation to clinical and endoscopic activity and outcome. *Eur.J.Gastroenterol.Hepatol.*, 17, 547-557.

Raddatz, D., Middel, P., Bockemuhl, M., Benohr, P., Wissmann, C., Schworer, H., Ramadori, G. (2004) Glucocorticoid receptor expression in inflammatory bowel disease: evidence for a mucosal down-regulation in steroid-unresponsive ulcerative colitis. *Aliment.Pharmacol.Ther.*, 19, 47-61.

Ravi, A., Garg, P., Sitaraman, S. V. (2007) Matrix metalloproteinases in inflammatory bowel disease: boon or a bane? *Inflamm.Bowel.Dis.*, 13, 97-107.

Roda, G., Caponi, A., Benevento, M., Nanni, P., Mezzanotte, L., Belluzzi, A., Mayer, L., Roda, A. (2010) New proteomic approaches for biomarker discovery in inflammatory bowel disease. *Inflamm.Bowel.Dis.*, 16, 1239-1246.

Roseth, A. G., Aadland, E., Grzyb, K. (2004) Normalization of faecal calprotectin: a predictor of mucosal healing in patients with inflammatory bowel disease. *Scand.J.Gastroenterol.*, 39, 1017-1020.

Roth, L. S., Chande, N., Ponich, T., Roth, M. L., Gregor, J. (2010) Predictors of disease severity in ulcerative colitis patients from Southwestern Ontario. *World J.Gastroenterol.*, 16, 232-236.

Sandborn, W. J. (1999) Severe Ulcerative Colitis. *Curr.Treat.Options.Gastroenterol.*, 2, 113-118.

Santos, A. C., Lopes, C., Guimaraes, J. T., Barros, H. (2005) Central obesity as a major determinant of increased high-sensitivity C-reactive protein in metabolic syndrome. *Int.J.Obes.(Lond)*, 29, 1452-1456.

Saverymuttu, S. H. (1986) Clinical remission in Crohn's disease--assessment using faecal 111In granulocyte excretion. *Digestion*, 33, 74-79.

Scaldaferri, F., Correale, C., Gasbarrini, A., Danese, S. (2010) Mucosal biomarkers in inflammatory bowel disease: key pathogenic players or disease predictors? *World J.Gastroenterol.*, 16, 2616-2625.

Schmidt, C., Giese, T., Hermann, E., Zeuzem, S., Meuer, S. C., Stallmach, A. (2007) Predictive value of mucosal TNF-alpha transcripts in steroid-refractory Crohn's disease patients receiving intensive immunosuppressive therapy. *Inflamm.Bowel.Dis.*, 13, 65-70.

Schreiber, S., Rutgeerts, P., Fedorak, R. N., Khaliq-Kareemi, M., Kamm, M. A., Boivin, M., Bernstein, C. N., Staun, M., Thomsen, O. O., Innes, A. (2005) A randomized, placebo-controlled trial of certolizumab pegol (CDP870) for treatment of Crohn's disease. *Gastroenterology*, 129, 807-818.

Schumacher, G. (1993) First attack of inflammatory bowel disease and infectious colitis. A clinical, histological and microbiological study with special reference to early diagnosis. *Scand.J.Gastroenterol.Suppl*, 198, 1-24.

Silberer, H., Kuppers, B., Mickisch, O., Baniewicz, W., Drescher, M., Traber, L., Kempf, A., Schmidt-Gayk, H. (2005) Fecal leukocyte proteins in inflammatory bowel disease and irritable bowel syndrome. *Clin.Lab*, 51, 117-126.

Solem, C. A., Loftus, E. V., Jr., Tremaine, W. J., Harmsen, W. S., Zinsmeister, A. R., Sandborn, W. J. (2005) Correlation of C-reactive protein with clinical, endoscopic, histologic, and radiographic activity in inflammatory bowel disease. *Inflamm.Bowel.Dis.*, 11, 707-712.

Strober, W., Zhang, F., Kitani, A., Fuss, I., Fichtner-Feigl, S. (2010) Proinflammatory cytokines underlying the inflammation of Crohn's disease. *Curr.Opin.Gastroenterol.*, 26, 310-317.

Tibble, J., Teahon, K., Thjodleifsson, B., Roseth, A., Sigthorsson, G., Bridger, S., Foster, R., Sherwood, R., Fagerhol, M., Bjarnason, I. (2000a) A simple method for assessing intestinal inflammation in Crohn's disease. *Gut*, 47, 506-513.

Tibble, J. A., Bjarnason, I. (2001) Fecal calprotectin as an index of intestinal inflammation. *Drugs Today (Barc.)*, 37, 85-96.

Tibble, J. A., Sigthorsson, G., Bridger, S., Fagerhol, M. K., Bjarnason, I. (2000b) Surrogate markers of intestinal inflammation are predictive of relapse in patients with inflammatory bowel disease. *Gastroenterology*, 119, 15-22.

Tibble, J. A., Sigthorsson, G., Foster, R., Forgacs, I., Bjarnason, I. (2002) Use of surrogate markers of inflammation and Rome criteria to distinguish organic from nonorganic intestinal disease. *Gastroenterology*, 123, 450-460.

Tibble, J. A., Sigthorsson, G., Foster, R., Scott, D., Fagerhol, M. K., Roseth, A., Bjarnason, I. (1999) High prevalence of NSAID enteropathy as shown by a simple faecal test. *Gut*, 45, 362-366.

Ton, H., Brandsnes, Dale, S., Holtlund, J., Skuibina, E., Schjonsby, H., Johne, B. (2000) Improved assay for fecal calprotectin. *Clin.Chim.Acta*, 292, 41-54.

Torres, M. I., Rios, A. (2008) Current view of the immunopathogenesis in inflammatory bowel disease and its implications for therapy. *World J.Gastroenterol.*, 14, 1972-1980.

Travis, S. P., Farrant, J. M., Ricketts, C., Nolan, D. J., Mortensen, N. M., Kettlewell, M. G., Jewell, D. P. (1996) Predicting outcome in severe ulcerative colitis. *Gut*, 38, 905-910.

Turner, D., Leach, S. T., Mack, D., Uusoue, K., McLernon, R., Hyams, J., Leleiko, N., Walters, T. D., Crandall, W., Markowitz, J., Otley, A. R., Griffiths, A. M., Day, A. S. (2010) Faecal calprotectin, lactoferrin, M2-pyruvate kinase and S100A12 in severe ulcerative colitis: a prospective multicentre comparison of predicting outcomes and monitoring response. *Gut*, 59, 1207-1212.

van Rheenen, P. F., Van, d., V, Fidler, V. (2010) Faecal calprotectin for screening of patients with suspected inflammatory bowel disease: diagnostic meta-analysis. *BMJ*, 341, c3369.

Vermeire, S., Peeters, M., Vlietinck, R., Joossens, S., Den, H. E., Bulteel, V., Bossuyt, X., Geypens, B., Rutgeerts, P. (2001) Anti-Saccharomyces cerevisiae antibodies (ASCA), phenotypes of IBD, and intestinal permeability: a study in IBD families. *Inflamm.Bowel.Dis.*, 7, 8-15.

Vermeire, S., Van, A. G., Rutgeerts, P. (2004) C-reactive protein as a marker for inflammatory bowel disease. *Inflamm.Bowel.Dis.*, 10, 661-665.

Vermeire, S., Van, A. G., Rutgeerts, P. (2006) Laboratory markers in IBD: useful, magic, or unnecessary toys? *Gut*, 55, 426-431.

Vernier, G., Sendid, B., Poulain, D., Colombel, J. F. (2004) Relevance of serologic studies in inflammatory bowel disease. *Curr.Gastroenterol.Rep.*, 6, 482-487.

Visser, M., Bouter, L. M., McQuillan, G. M., Wener, M. H., Harris, T. B. (1999) Elevated C-reactive protein levels in overweight and obese adults. *JAMA*, 282, 2131-2135.

Visser, M., Bouter, L. M., McQuillan, G. M., Wener, M. H., Harris, T. B. (2001) Low-grade systemic inflammation in overweight children. *Pediatrics*, 107, E13.

von Roon, A. C., Karamountzos, L., Purkayastha, S., Reese, G. E., Darzi, A. W., Teare, J. P., Paraskeva, P., Tekkis, P. P. (2007) Diagnostic precision of fecal calprotectin for inflammatory bowel disease and colorectal malignancy. *Am.J.Gastroenterol.*, 102, 803-813.

von, L. B., Barthel, B., Coupland, S. E., Riecken, E. O., Rosewicz, S. (2000) Differential expression of matrix metalloproteinases and their tissue inhibitors in colon mucosa of patients with inflammatory bowel disease. *Gut*, 47, 63-73.

Wagner, M., Peterson, C. G., Ridefelt, P., Sangfelt, P., Carlson, M. (2008) Fecal markers of inflammation used as surrogate markers for treatment outcome in relapsing inflammatory bowel disease. *World J.Gastroenterol.*, 14, 5584-5589.

Walker, L. J., Aldhous, M. C., Drummond, H. E., Smith, B. R., Nimmo, E. R., Arnott, I. D., Satsangi, J. (2004) Anti-Saccharomyces cerevisiae antibodies (ASCA) in Crohn's disease are associated with disease severity but not NOD2/CARD15 mutations. *Clin.Exp.Immunol.*, 135, 490-496.

Zimmerman, N. P., Vongsa, R. A., Wendt, M. K., Dwinell, M. B. (2008) Chemokines and chemokine receptors in mucosal homeostasis at the intestinal epithelial barrier in inflammatory bowel disease. *Inflamm.Bowel.Dis.*, 14, 1000-1011.

6

Polysaccharides for Colon–Targeted Drug Delivery: Improved Drug–Release Specificity and Therapeutic Benefits

Annette Hartzell and Devin J. Rose
University of Nebraska- Lincoln
United States of America

1. Introduction

Ulcerative colitis (UC) is a chronic, immunologically-mediated disorder which affects the gastrointestinal tract. This disease is characterized by inflammation of the colonic or rectal mucosa, leading to rectal bleeding, diarrhea, and abdominal pain. UC, along with Crohn's disease, is referred to as inflammatory bowel disease. The specific cause of this disease is unknown, but research has suggested that it is most likely initiated by a combination of host susceptibility and environmental triggers. These factors lead to an overly-aggressive T-cell response to bacteria in the gastrointestinal tract. An abnormal ratio between beneficial and detrimental microbes in the gut may also contribute to the development of this disease, as well as defects in the function of the intestinal mucosal barrier. No medical cure has been developed for UC; treatment focuses on inducing and maintaining remission (Sartor, 2006).

Anti-inflammatory drugs, particularly those that contain 5-aminosalicylic acid (5-ASA), are often used to treat UC. The effectiveness of these aminosalicylate drugs is related to their mucosal concentration. Because free 5-ASA is rapidly absorbed in the small intestine, this drug must be encapsulated or conjugated to be effectively delivered to the colon. Methods for colonic delivery of 5-ASA include chemically attaching it to a carrier molecule or encapsulating it with pH or time-release polymers, but these methods exhibit various limitations (Caprilli et al., 2009).

The use of polysaccharides as conjugate or encapsulation materials has been explored as a means of targeting the delivery of 5-ASA to the colon. The purpose of this chapter is to discuss approaches to using polysaccharides as colon-targeted drug delivery systems, and to discuss how using polysaccharides in these drug formulations may provide therapeutic benefits beyond drug delivery.

1.1 Aminosalicylates in UC treatment

Aminosalicylates were the first drugs that were shown to be effective against UC. The first of this class of drugs was sulphasalazine. At the time of this drug's development, it was thought that both rheumatoid arthritis and UC were caused by streptococcal infection and that UC symptoms began in the connective tissue of the submucosa. Sulphasalazine was developed by combining sulphapyridine, which was effective against bacteria, with 5-ASA, which was active on connective tissue. Sulphasalazine was shown to improve both rheumatoid arthritis and UC. At the recommended dose of 500mg 4 to 6 times per day, however, approximately 15 to 20% of patients experienced side effects such as headaches, nausea, vomiting, fever, cyanosis, allergic reactions, jaundice, leucopenia and agranulcytosis (Caprilli et al., 2009). Later research demonstrated that 5-ASA was the part of sulphasalazine responsible for the drug's therapeutic effects against UC. Enemas of sulphasalazine, 5-ASA and sulphapyridine were given to patients with UC. Improvement was seen in only 5% of patients receiving sulphapyridine, as opposed to 30% of those receiving either sulphasalazine or 5-ASA (Azad Khan et al., 1977). This discovery paved the way for other 5-ASA-containing drugs developed for the treatment of UC. Today, aminosalicylates are still the standard therapy for the induction and maintenance of remission in UC patients (Hanauer, 2004).

1.2 Mechanism of therapeutic action of aminosalicylate-containing drugs

Aminosalicylate drugs are able to decrease the symptoms of UC, although the exact mechanism by which they act is unknown. Aminosalicylates have a demonstrated inhibitory effect on pro-inflammatory mediators released by the colonic and rectal mucosa. 5-ASA can interact with the peroxisome proliferator activated receptor γ, which acts to inhibit the mucosal production of inflammatory cytokines (Caprilli et al., 2009). 5-ASA also exhibits antioxidant properties, and can act as a free radical scavenger (Osterman & Lichtenstein, 2009).

Aminosalicylates act at the site of inflammation topically; the effectiveness of 5-ASA-containing drugs is linked directly to their mucosal concentration. Therefore, it is necessary that aminosalicylates be delivered effectively to the colon. Delivery can be performed by administering the drug rectally or orally. When free 5-ASA is delivered orally, however, it is absorbed in the upper gastrointestinal tract, and does not reach the colon. Therefore, the drug must be protected in some way in order to ensure that it is delivered to the colon effectively (Caprilli et al., 2009).

2. Current 5-aminosalicylic acid formulations: Varieties and limitations

There are currently four main methods of orally delivering 5-ASA to the colon. These methods are through diazo compounds, pH-dependent formulations, time-controlled release, and a multi-matrix system (Table 1).

In the first method, 5-ASA is attached to a carrier molecule by a diazo bond, which is then split by bacteria in the gastrointestinal tract. Commercial drugs of this type are known as Olsalazine, Balsalazide, and Sulphasalazine (Table 1). Sulphasalazine has been associated with numerous side effects, as explained, while Olsalazine and Balsalazide have not been shown to cause side effects (Sandborn, 2006a).

The pH dependent release system involves an acid-resistant acrylic resin known as Eudragit-s. The acrylic protects the 5-ASA during its passage through the gastrointestinal tract, but is dissolved in the alkaline environment of the colon, releasing the 5-ASA (Dew et al., 1982). Asacol is a commercial drug of this variety. A limitation of this delivery system is that a high degree of variation exists in the pH levels of the gastrointestinal tracts of different individuals, especially for those who are in a diseased state. Also, pH differences between the distal ileum, cecum and proximal colon are small. Therefore, it is difficult to determine exactly where in the gastrointestinal tract the 5-ASA will be released (Hanauer, 2004).

Formulation	Example	Site of release	Unit (g)	Dose (g/d)		Limitations
				Active	Remission	
Conjugated						
5-ASA linked to sulfapyrazine by azo bond	Sulfasalazine	Colon	0.5	2-6	2-4	Diarrhea
5-ASA dimer linked by azo-bond	Olsalazine	Colon	0.5	Not effective	1	
5-ASA linked to 4-amino-benzoyl-β-alanine by azo bond	Balsalazide	Colon	0.75	4.6-7.5	4	
Encapsulated						
Eudragit-S coated tablets	Asacol	Ileum, colon	0.4	1.6-4.8	0.8-1.6	No large change in pH from ileum to colon; pH differences among individuals
Ethylcellulose-coated micro-granules (time-release)	Pentasa	Small intestine, colon	0.25-1.0	2-4	4	Variations in transit time
Eudragit-L-coated pellets with additional retarding polymer in the pellet core	Mesalamine pellets	Ileum, colon	0.5	1.5-4.5	Not studied	
Eudragit-S-coated tablets with lipophilic and hydrophilic matrices in the tablet core	Lialda	Ileum, colon	1.2	2.4-4.8	Not studied	

Table 1. Aminosalicylate drugs: Examples, limitations, and doses (Sandborn, 2006b; Caprilli et al., 2009)

The time-controlled release system uses a microsphere of ethylcellulose to coat the 5-ASA. The microsphere swells and dissolves slowly as the drug moves through the gastrointestinal tract, releasing the 5-ASA mainly in the duodenum and proximal colon (Rasmussen et al., 1982). Pentasa is the commercial name for this delivery system. As for the pH dependent release system, the major limitation of this drug type lies in patient variation. The time it takes for the drug to travel through the gastrointestinal tract can vary from person to person, leading to a non-specific point of drug release. Moreover, in patients with UC, transit time through the colon can be accelerated, leading to incomplete drug release (Jain et al., 2007).

The newest delivery system developed for 5-ASA is the multimatrix, or MMX system. In this formulation, 5-ASA microparticles are trapped within a lipophilic matrix, which is then dispersed throughout a hydrophilic matrix. This tablet core is then coated with an acid-resistant polymer, which dissolves when the pH is above 7.0. When delivered via the MMX system, the 5-ASA is released beginning in the terminal ileum. This delivery system allows for slow release of 5-ASA along the length of the colon and rectum (Caprilli et al., 2009).

One limitation common to all of the drugs currently used to treat UC is the high dose needed to achieve therapeutic results (Table 1). Because the common dose of these aminosalicylate drugs is 225 to 500 mg per dose, patients may have to take over 10 pills per day in order to treat their conditions. This high pill burden often leads to low compliance rates among patients (Osterman & Lichtenstein, 2009).

All formulations of 5-ASA are metabolized to N-acetyl-5-ASA by the same pathway. A meta-analysis looking at the fecal and systemic (urinary) excretion of N-acetyl-5-ASA using various formulations was carried out. A wide range of excretion amounts was found for each 5-ASA formulation, due to differences in study designs. However, a clear trend was spotted in regard to fecal vs. urinary excretion, based upon whether the patients in the studies had active or quiescent colitis. It was found that patients with active colitis had higher levels of 5-ASA in their feces, while those in remission had higher urinary levels of the drug. This is because UC causes a decrease in transit time through the gastrointestinal tract, providing less time for 5-ASA to be absorbed (Hanauer, 2004). Therefore, higher doses of 5-ASA are required to treat active UC, in comparison to amounts required to maintain remission (Table 1).

3. Polysaccharides for colon-targeted drug delivery

The use of various polysaccharides has been explored as a means of colon-targeted drug delivery. Polysaccharides provide several benefits as carrier molecules or encapsulation materials. They generally have a predictable degradation pattern, allowing for consistent release of the drug from the encapsulation matrix. Polysaccharide matrices also hydrate and swell as they travel through the gastrointestinal tract, creating a barrier against diffusion of the drug. When they arrive at the colon, colonic bacteria and enzymes are able to degrade the polysaccharide matrices to release the encapsulated drug (Wong et al., 2011). Polysaccharides also exist with a wide variety of functional groups, molecular weights, and chemical compositions. Some have a high stability to temperature and heat, while also having high biodegradability and low toxicity. Many polysaccharides are approved as pharmaceutical excipients (Jain et al., 2007).

Polysaccharides have been shown to be useful carrier systems for the delivery of aminosalicylates, in both encapsulation matrices and as conjugate carrier molecules. The rate of drug release can be tailored by controlling the polysaccharide carrier used and the method of preparation of the final 5-ASA-polysaccharide product (Wong et al., 2011).

3.1 Encapsulation polysaccharides

Several polysaccharides have been used successfully as encapsulation materials for aminosalicylate drugs, and are discussed below.

3.1.1 Starch

Enteric-coated starch capsules have been studied for the colon-targeted delivery of aminosalicylic acid. In one study, 5-ASA was placed into starch capsules produced by injection moulding, which were then covered with a Eudragit coating. The capsules were evaluated over time for capsule disintegration and drug release in gastric and intestinal media. The capsules were found to be stable in the gastric environment, but were disintegrated between one and two hours following immersion in the intestinal medium (Vilivalam et al., 2000). Another study by the same authors compared the release time of 5-ASA from 5-ASA beads manufactured by extrusion-spheronization. 5-ASA beads in an uncoated starch capsule and 5-ASA beads in an enteric-coated starch capsule yielded similar time release results, but the 5-ASA in the coated starch capsule had the largest lag time in 5-ASA release (Vilivalam et al., 2000).

The amylose portion of starch has also been studied for use as a coating for the delivery of 5-ASA to the colon, and similar results were seen as in the starch coating studies. A resin made of a combination of amylose and ethyl cellulose was used to coat 5-ASA pellets. The coated drug was stable in simulated gastric and small intestine solutions for 12 hours. The 5-ASA was released within 4 hours when placed in a simulated colonic environment (Milojevic et al., 1996).

3.1.2 Pectin

Pectins are polysaccharides consisting of (1→4)-linked α-D-galacturonic acid with intermittent (1→2)-linked α-L-rhamnose units along the backbone with side chains of varying complexity containing galacturonic acid, galactose, rhamnose, arabinose, and other sugars. Most drug delivery studies use commercial pectin, which contains very few side chains (as these are removed during processing and purification). Backbone galacturonic acid units carry with them varying degrees of methylation. Low methyl esterified pectins can cross-link with divalent cations, which is important in encapsulation for drug delivery. Pectins are naturally resistant to gastric and small intestinal enzymes, but are degraded by colonic bacterial enzymes. They are soluble in water, which is a hurdle in the development of pectin-based drug delivery systems. This challenge can be overcome, however, through the choice of pectin type, the use of additives, or the use of accompanying hydrophobic polymers such as ethylcellulose (Jain et al., 2007).

Pectins have been used successfully as matrix materials in several studies (Jain et al., 2007). For example, a pectin matrix cross-linked by calcium ions has been used to successfully deliver chemotherapy drugs to the colon (Wong et al., 2011). Another study found that a compression coat of high methoxy pectin was able to protect a core tablet during mouth to colon transit. The *in vitro* portion of this study showed that the pectin coat was able to protect the tablet under gastric conditions. *In vivo* scintigraphic (radioactive tracing) results confirmed this, and also showed that the pectin-coated tablets dissolved once they reached the colon (Ashford et al., 1993). A mixture of pectin and chitosan has been shown to give protective results similar to a pectin coating, but with a lower coat weight (Fernandez-Hervas, 1998).

3.1.3 Inulin

Inulin is a fructan consisting of 2 to 60 (2→1)-linked β-D-fructose units, with glucose often as the initial moiety of the chain. It is a storage polysaccharide which is found in many plants, including onion, garlic, artichoke and chicory. Inulin is resistant to degradation in the upper gastrointestinal tract, but is preferentially fermented by *Bifidobacteria* in the colon (Jain et al., 2007).

Inulin has been incorporated into Eudragit RS films, which are able to resist degradation in the upper gastrointestinal tract, but are metabolized by beneficial bacteria in the colon. Hydrogels of inulin have also been developed, in which vinyl groups are attached to inulin chains by free radical polymerization to induce intramolecular cross-linking (Van den Mooter et al., 2003). Methacrylated inulin has also been used as a hydrogel for targeted drug delivery. An *in vitro* stability study demonstrated that the higher the degree of substitution of the hydrogels, the more resistant they were to degradation by inulinase (Jain et al., 2007).

3.1.4 Galactomannan-containing gums

Galactomannan-containing gums have also been used as encapsulation materials for colon-targeted drug delivery. One such gum is guar gum, which is obtained from the endosperm of *Cyamposis tetragonolobus*. It is comprised of a mannan backbone with galactose side chains. Guar gum can be used to coat colon-bound drugs by compression, retarding their release. The guar gum is then degraded in the large intestine by microbial enzymes, releasing the drug (Jain et al., 2007).

Alternatively guar gum can used to encapsulate drugs through derivatization of the hydroxyl groups. In one study, guar gum was substituted with carboxymethyl groups, which were then cross-linked with barium ion. This was used as a microencapsulation matrix for a model compound: bovine serum albumin. Very little of the drug was released when the capsules were exposed to a pH of 1.2, simulating the stomach, but the drug was released in a pH of 7.4., simulating the large intestine. The researchers concluded that this formulation would be useful for gastrointestinal drug delivery (Thimma & Tammishetti, 2001).

Locust bean gum has also been used as an encapsulation material. Locust bean gum is derived from carob seeds, and is also a mannan with galactose side chains, though less branched then guar gum. In one study, locust bean gum was combined with chitosan in the ratios of 2:3, 3:2, and 4:1. The locust bean gum/chitosan mixture was applied to 5-ASA cores, which were created by tablet pressing and the stability of the formulation was tested *in vitro* and *in vivo*. The results of both studies showed that this coating was able to protect the drug from being released in the stomach and small intestine, but was degraded by colonic bacterial enzymes (Raghavan et al., 2002).

The galactomannans in locust bean gum can be cross-linked, forming a water-insoluble film, which can then be degraded by bacteria in the colon (Hirsch et al., 1995). Locust bean gum galactomannans were crosslinked by 1,4-butanedioldiglycidyl ether, yielding a low crosslinked product that can be used to form films. The crosslinked galactomannans were incubated anaerobically with the contents of a fresh pig cecum, representing the human colonic microflora, and degraded within 270 minutes. The material was then used to spray-coat theophylline tablets, which were used as a model drug. When placed under conditions representing passage through the small intestine, drug release was observed, but the researchers concluded that the lag time prior to drug release could be increased by applying a thicker coating of the crosslinked galactomannans (Hirsch et al., 1995).

3.1.5 Alginates

Alginates, which are derived from seaweed, have not been used as an encapsulation material, but have been utilized as a core for aminosalicylate drugs. Alginates consist of (1→4) linked β-D-mannuronic acid and α-L-glucuronic acid residues. Alginates are able to form gels in the presence of divalent cations (Jain et al., 2007). In one study, calcium alginate beads were formed through the drop-wise addition of sodium alginate into a solution of calcium chloride. 5-ASA was spray coated on the calcium alginate beads and coated by pH-dependent and time-released polymers. As the drug coated beads moved through the gastrointestinal tract, the calcium alginate beads swelled until they burst through the outer coatings due to an osmotic gradient, releasing the 5-ASA. This delivery system allows the 5-ASA to be delivered to the ileum (Lin & Ayres, 1992).

3.2 Conjugate polysaccharides

In addition to their use as encapsulation materials, polysaccharides have been used as conjugate carrier molecules for the delivery of 5-ASA to the colon. The polysaccharides can be attached either to the carboxyl group or the amino group of the 5-ASA. Conjugates prepared by these methods have been shown to survive conditions in the stomach and small intestine and are able to reach the colon intact. In the colon, the 5-ASA is cleaved from the carrier molecule through the action of bacterial azo-reductases, esterases, and glycoside hydrolases.

3.2.1 Dextran

Dextrans are a class of polysaccharides consisting of linear chains of α-D glucose molecules. Ninety five percent of the chains have glucose linked (1→6), while the side chains are linked (1→3). Dextrans are obtained from lactobacilli organisms. *Bacteriodes* in the gastrointestinal tract produce dextranase enzymes, which are capable of cleaving dextran chains (Jain et al., 2007).

Dextrans have been used as carrier molecules for 5-ASA in several studies. In one study, dextrans were oxidized using sodium periodate. The aldehyde groups of the dextrans were then attached to the α-amino group of 5-ASA. Dextrans were oxidized by incubating them with different amounts of $NaIO_4$. The amount of $NaIO_4$ consumed was determined by back titration. The more $NaIO_4$ consumed, the more oxidized the dextrans were considered to be. Degree of substitution was defined as the mg of 5-ASA per 100 mg of total product. Degrees of substitution between 15 and 50 were obtained, depending on the degree of oxidation of the dextran. It was found that dextrans with a high degree of oxidation gave the maximum degree of conjugation to 5-ASA, but were then resistant to hydrolysis by dextranase. Less oxidized dextran bound a lower amount of 5-ASA, but were more able to be digested by dextranase, making them better candidates for carrier molecules (Ahmad et al., 2006). In another study, dextran prodrugs of 5-ASA were created by linking the dextran to the carboxyl group of the 5-ASA via an ester linkage. The conjugates were incubated with small intestinal and caecal contents of rats. It was found that no 5-ASA was released during the incubation with the intestinal contents, but incubation with the caecal contents induced drug release (Jung et al., 1998).

3.2.2 Cyclodextrins

Cyclodextrins are cyclic oligosaccharides which are made up of six to eight α-D-glucose units joined through (1→4) glycosidic bonds (Jain et al., 2007). There are three forms of cyclodextrins α-Cyclodextrin is a six-membered ring, β-cyclodextrin is a seven-membered ring, and γ-cyclodextrin is an eight-membered ring. Cyclodextrins are able to resist digestion in the stomach and small intestine, but are fermented in the colon. The interior of a cyclodextrin molecule is lipophilic, while the exterior is hydrophilic. This allows the cyclodextrins to form inclusion complexes with hydrophobic drugs (Zou et al., 2005).

5-ASA was linked to α, β, and γ cyclodextrins through an ester linkage to the carboxyl group of the 5-ASA. The degree of substitution, or the percent of hydroxyl groups containing 5-ASA, was measured. The impact of degree of substitution on the release of 5-ASA from cyclodextrin was also evaluated. It was found that cyclodextrins with degrees of substitution less than 30% provided the greatest release of 5-ASA in the caecal and colonic environment (Zou et al., 2005).

4. Therapeutic agents as carrier molecules

Using a therapeutic agent, rather than an inert compound, as the carrier molecule may improve the effectiveness of aminosalicylate drugs. Several polysaccharides have been shown to protect against UC inflammation, making them ideal candidates for carrier molecules (Ewaschuk, 2006). These polysaccharides can be incorporated into films, cross-linked, or conjugated through ester linkages.

There are several benefits of using polysaccharides as therapeutic carrier molecules. For one, drugs can be selectively released in the colon by bacterial esterases, rather than relying on gradual changes in pH or highly variable time release. Using polysaccharides can also allow for prolonged release of the drug in the distal colon, which is the site of most UC inflammation. The rate of release is dependent on the structure of the polysaccharide, as well as the activity of the bacterial esterases. Because polysaccharides have therapeutic benefits against UC, using them as carrier molecules might allow for a decrease in drug dosage requirements. On a lower dose of drugs, patients would likely experience fewer side effects, and patient compliance rates would increase. A polysaccharide carrier system would also increase the water solubility of the drugs. Increased solubility would allow for the administration of larger doses of the drug in beverage form, rather than in pills, which would also increase patient compliance.

5. Therapeutic benefits for polysaccharides against UC

Many of the polysaccharides described above are classified as dietary fibers. Dietary fiber encompasses a number of plant substances which are resistant to hydrolysis by digestive enzymes in the small bowel. This includes non-starch polysaccharides, resistant starch, cellulose, hemicellulose, oligosaccharides, pectins, gums, lignin, and waxes (James et al., 2003).

When dietary fibers reach the large intestine, they are fermented by gut bacteria. In general, soluble dietary fiber is fermentable by colonic bacteria, producing short chain fatty acids, while insoluble fiber is poorly fermentable (Galvez et al., 2005). Different carbohydrate substrates produce different ratios of short chain fatty acids (SCFA). For example, resistant starch (RS) is butyrogenic, guar gum and psyllium are mainly propiogenic, while pectin is acetogenic (Rose & Hamaker, 2011).

SCFA have many effects in the gastrointestinal tract. For example, SCFAs lower the pH of the lumen of the large bowel. This prevents the growth of some pathogenic bacteria. Butyrate, especially, is important for the maintenance of colonic health. Butyrate has been shown to prevent colonic inflammation by inhibiting NF-κB activation (Inan et al., 2000). Butyrate may also help to prevent colon cancer, by playing a role in the repair of damaged DNA, and the induction of apoptosis in transformed epithelial cells (Lührs et al., 2002).

In addition to producing SCFA, many polysaccharides are prebiotics. Prebiotics are food substances that are not digested in the small intestine and promote the growth of certain beneficial species of bacteria in the colon (Gibson et al., 2004). Prebiotics such as lactulose, fructo-oligosaccharides (FOS), inulin, psyllium, and germinated barley foodstuffs have been shown to stimulate the growth and metabolism of protective bacteria endogenous to the human gut (Ewaschuk & Dieleman, 2006). These protective bacteria can secrete metabolites that can help to reduce the amount of pro-inflammatory factors produced by the colonic mucosa. Bacteria that are thought to be beneficial to gut health include *Lactobacilli, Bifidobacterium breve, Streptococcus thermophiles, B. bifidum, and Ruminococcus* (Ewaschuk & Dieleman, 2006). Many of the carbohydrate carrier molecules discussed above are prebiotics, which stimulate the growth of these protective bacteria.

5.1 *Plantago ovata* (psyllium) seeds

Plantago ovata seeds, commonly known as psyllium, have been tested as remission maintenance treatments in UC. Psyllium seeds include a complex glucuronoarabinoxylan that is composed of a β-(1→3 or →4)-D-Xyl*p* backbone, with arabinoxylan, xylose, glucuronic acid and galactose side chains (Rose & Hamaker, 2011). One of the earliest studies looked at the effects of ingesting psyllium husks on quiescent UC patients. The researchers found that the psyllium husks were effective in reducing UC symptoms in these patients. Patients on the psyllium husk treatment reported decreased symptoms such as bloating, diarrhoea, and abdominal pain. The researchers hypothesized that the therapeutic benefit was primarily a result of the fiber's normalizing effect on transit time through the bowel. Also, because psyllium husks are mainly composed of soluble fermentable fiber, their fermentation in the ascending colon would cause an increase in SCFA production, possibly leading to further health benefits (Hallert et al., 1991).

In another study, UC patients in remission were given 5-ASA, psyllium seed (which contains dietary fiber) or a combination of the two. No difference in disease states were observed between any of the treatment groups. This indicates that psyllium seed might be as effective a treatment for maintaining the remission of UC as the 5-ASA drug mesalamine.

This study also showed an increase in SCFA production in patients receiving psyllium (Fernandez-Banares et al., 1999).

Plantago ovata seeds have also been shown to be therapeutic against an induced animal model of UC. Colitis was induced in rats via an enema containing 2,4,6,-trinitrobenzene sulfonic acid (TNBS). There were 3 experimental groups; a non-colitic group, a colitic group which received a standard diet, and a colitic group which was fed a standard diet supplemented with psyllium seeds. Rats which received dietary fiber supplementation showed lower inflammation histologically, and had lower levels of myeloperoxidase, tumor necrosis factor α, and nitric oxide synthase activity, some of the mediators involved in the inflammatory response (Rodriguez et al., 2002).

5.1.1 Germinated barley foodstuff

Germinated barley foodstuff (GBF) is made up of the aleurone layer and the scutellum fraction of brewer's spent grain. GBF is comprised primarily of dietary fiber, in the form of low-lignified hemicellulose, and glutamine-rich protein. The dietary fiber portion of GBF is efficiently fermented by beneficial colonic bacteria such as *Bifodobacterium* and *Lactobacillus,* which increases the concentration of SCFA, especially butyrate, in the colonic lumen (Galvez et al., 2005).

Several studies have examined the effects of GBF on patients with UC. In one study, patients with mild to moderately active UC were administered a conventional anti-inflammatory treatment, either with or without the addition of GBF. After 4 weeks on these regimens, patients who had GBF added to their treatment showed a significant decrease in clinical activity scores as compared to those who were on the conventional treatment only. There were no side effects observed with the GBF treatment, and faecal concentrations of the beneficial gut bacteria *Bifidobacterium* and *Eubacterium limosum* were increased (Kanauchi et al., 2002). An earlier study which also used GBF as a supplementation to traditional anti-inflammatory treatment obtained similar results (Mitsuyama et al., 1998). Notably, this study found that inflammation significantly increased within 4 weeks of halting the GBF supplementation (Mitsuyama et al., 1998).

Additionally, GBF can be used as a maintenance therapy to help maintain UC remission. When given to quiescent patients daily, in conjunction with traditional treatments, GBF was correlated with a reduction in UC symptoms. The rate of UC relapse was also lower in the group receiving GBF in addition to standard maintenance therapy (Hanai et al., 2004).

GBF has been shown to be effective in an animal model of UC. Kanauchi et al. (2003) demonstrated that GBF was therapeutic in treating mice with dextran sodium sulphate (DSS)-induced colitis. Mice were divided in to two groups and fed either a control diet of cellulose, or a diet containing GBF. After one week on each diet, experimental colitis was induced by adding 2% DSS to their drinking water, and the mice were sacrificed 6 days later. The researchers found that mice that had been on the GBF diet showed significantly lower disease activity, weight loss, and inflammatory disease markers.

5.1.2 Resistant starch

RS is defined as starch and starch products which escape digestion in the human small intestine, acting as dietary fiber. In the large bowel RS is highly fermentable and contributes greatly to colonic SCFA production. There are a number of types of RS: RS1 (physically inaccessibly starch), RS2a (uncooked starch), RS2b (high amylose starch), RS3 (retrograded starch), and RS4 (chemically modified starch). Some studies have demonstrated reduced postprandial glucose and insulin responses in patients who were fed RS. In animal models, RS has been shown to decrease serum lipid and cholesterol concentrations, although no such effect has been conclusively demonstrated in humans (Rose & Hamaker, 2010).

RS has been shown to be therapeutic in an experimental animal model of colitis. Colitis was induced in rats via a TNBS enema. The animals were fed standard diets either with or without the addition of granular pea starch (a source of RS2). They were sacrificed between 3 and 21 days after the induction of colitis, and the colons of the rats were examined. Rats which were fed diets including RS had an increased uptake of SCFA, and higher luminal concentrations of beneficial gut bacteria (Jacobasch et al., 1999).

5.2 Lactulose

Lactulose is a non-digestible disaccharide comprised of fructose and galactose produced by alkali isomerisation of lactose. It is not a common dietary carbohydrate, but is used in the pharmaceutical industry for the treatment of hepatic encephalopathy and constipation. It is a prebiotic carbohydrate, which is selectively digested by bacteria in the cecum and colon.

Lactulose was proposed as a possible treatment for UC based upon its demonstrated ability to clear infectious bacteria and bacterial endotoxins from the gastrointestinal tract (Liao et al., 1994). Lactulose was then tested for efficacy in treating a DSS-induced mouse model of colitis (Rumi et al., 2004). In this study, colitis was induced in the mice through the addition of DSS to their drinking water over a period of 7 days. The mice were then treated orally with lactulose twice daily for 6 days. Compared to control animals, mice treated with lactulose exhibited decreased UC symptoms such as colonic ulceration and myeloperoxidase activity. The prebiotic properties of lactulose are believed to be responsible for its therapeutic potential in treating UC (Rumi et al,. 2004).

5.3 Fructooligosaccharides and inulin

FOS are composed of (1→2)-linked β-D-fructose units, with a terminal glucose unit (Rose & Hamaker 2011). FOS are resistant to digestion in the small intestine, and are fermented in the colon by gut bacteria (Le Blay et al., 1999). In one study, FOS were administered to rats with TNBS-induced colitis through intragastric infusions at a level of 1g/day for two weeks. The FOS were found to decrease the rats' gross inflammation score, myeloperoxidase activity and pH, and to increase the lactate, butyrate, and lactic acid-producing bacteria concentrations. The therapeutic effects of FOS are thought to be primarily due to their ability to increase lactic acid-producing bacteria counts in the intestine (Cherbut et al,. 2003). In contrast, Moreau et al. (2007) showed that FOS were ineffective in improving DSS-induced colitis in rats, as compared with RS. The differences between the effects of these two carbohydrates could be due to differences in SCFA and pH profiles produced through bacterial fermentation in the colon.

Inulin is the same basic structure as FOS, except includes longer chain fractions (up to 60 units). Inulin is a prebiotic, and has been shown to be effective in treating UC. Inulin has been demonstrated to improve the symptoms of DSS-induced UC in a rat model. Rats with

DSS-induced colitis received inulin either orally or through an enema. Inulin given through an oral route was shown to decrease inflammation in the rats, while the inulin given via enema had no effect (Videla et al., 2001).

In a human clinical study, oligofructose-enriched inulin, which is a 50:50 mixture of FOS and long-chain inulin, was shown to alleviate inflammation associated with UC. The patients had been in remission with either 5-ASA maintenance or without any drug, and had experienced a relapse of their UC. The patients were treated with a combination of 5-ASA and oligofructose-enriched inulin or a placebo for a period of two weeks. Fecal calprotectin was measured as a marker of inflammation. Patients who received the oligofructose-enriched inulin showed lower fecal calprotectin levels than the control group, indicating that oligofructose-enriched inulin is able to reduce inflammation from UC (Casellas et al., 2007).

6. Conclusions

This chapter has discussed the use of polysaccharides for colon-targeted drug delivery. Polysaccharides offer several advantages over traditional colon-targeted drug delivery systems. For instance, polysaccharides are natural polymers with no toxicity. Furthermore, the variation in structure and mode of conjugation/encapsulation could lead to improved site-specific drug release, reducing the need for excessive amounts of the drug. Finally, polysaccharides may lead to reduction in disease severity beyond that provided by the drug due to fermentation of the polysaccharide by bacteria. In this way, the polysaccharides not only act as carrier molecules, but as therapeutic agents as well.

7. References

Ahmad, S., Tester, R. F., Corbett, A., & Karkalas, J. (2006). Dextran and 5-aminosalicylic acid (5-ASA) conjugates: synthesis, characterisation and enzymic hydrolysis. *Carbohydrate research*, 341, 16, pp. (2694-2701), ISSN: 0008-6215.

Ashford, M., Fell, J., Attwood, D., Sharma, H., & Woodhead, P. (1993). An evaluation of pectin as a carrier for drug targeting to the colon. *Journal of Controlled Release*, 26, 3, pp. (213-220), ISSN: 0168-3659.

Azad Khan, A. K., Piris, J., & Truelove, S. C. (1977). An experiment to determine the active therapeutic moiety of sulphasalazine. *Lancet*, 2, 8044, pp. (892-895), doi: 10.1016/S0140-6736(77)90831-5.

Caprilli, R., Cesarini, M., Angelucci, E., & Frieri, G. (2009). The long journey of salicylates in ulcerative colitis: The past and the future. *Journal of Crohn's and Colitis*, 3, 3, pp. (149–156). doi: 18773-9946.

Casellas, F., Borruel, N., Torrejón, A., Varela, E., Antolin, M., Guarner, F., & Malagelada, J. R. (2007). Oral oligofructose-enriched inulin supplementation in acute ulcerative colitis is well tolerated and associated with lowered faecal calprotectin. *Alimentary Pharmacology & Therapeutics*, 25,9, pp. (1061-1067), ISSN: 0269-2813.

Cherbut, C., Michel, C., & Lecannu, G. (2003). The prebiotic characteristics of fructooligosaccharides are necessary for reduction of TNBS-induced colitis in rats. *The Journal of Nutrition*, 133,1, pp. (21-27), ISSN: 0022-3166.

Dew, M. J., Hughes, P., Harries, A. D., Williams, G., Evans, B. K., & Rhodes, J. (1982). Maintenance of remission in ulcerative colitis with oral preparation of 5-aminosalicylic acid. *British Medical Journal (Clinical research ed.)*, 285, 6347, pp. (1012), doi: 10.1136/bmj.285.6355.

Ewaschuk, J. B., & Dieleman, L. A. (2006). Probiotics and prebiotics in chronic inflammatory bowel diseases. *World Journal of Gastroenterology : WJG*, 12, 37, pp. (5941-5950), ISSN: 1007-9327.

Fernandez-Banares, F., Hinojosa, J., Sanchez-Lombrana, J., Navarro, E., Martinez-Salmeron, J., Garcia-Puges, A., Gonzalez-Huix, F., Riera, J., Gonzalez-Lara, V., Dominguez-Abascal, F., Gine, J. J., Moles, J. Gollomon, F., & Gassull, M. A.. (1999). Randomized clinical trial of Plantago ovata seeds(dietary fiber) as compared with mesalamine in maintaining remission in ulcerative colitis. *The American Journal of Gastroenterology*, 94 ,2, pp. (427–433), ISSN: 0002-9270.

Fernández-Hervás, M. (1998). Pectin/chitosan mixtures as coatings for colon-specific drug delivery: an in vitro evaluation. *International Journal of Pharmaceutics*, 169, 1, pp. (115-119), ISSN: 0378-5173.

Galvez, J., Rodríguez-Cabezas, M. E., & Zarzuelo, A. (2005). Effects of dietary fiber on inflammatory bowel disease. *Molecular Nutrition & Food Research*, 49 ,6, pp. (601-608), ISSN: 1613-4125.

Gibson, G. R., Probert, H. M., Loo, J. V., Rastall, R. a, & Roberfroid, M. B. (2004). Dietary modulation of the human colonic microbiota: updating the concept of prebiotics. *Nutrition Research Reviews*, 17, 2, pp. (259-275), ISSN: 0954-4224.

Hallert, C., Kaldma, M., & Petersson, B. G. (1991). Ispaghula husk may relieve gastrointestinal symptoms in ulcerative colitis in remission. *Scandinavian Journal of Gastroenterology*, 26, 7, pp. (747-750), ISSN: 0036-5521.

Hanai, H., Kanauchi, Osamu, Mitsuyama, Keiichi, Andoh, A., Takeuchi, Ken, Takayuki, I., Araki, Y., Fujiyama, Y., Toyonaga, A., Sata, M., Kojima, A., Fukuda, M., Bamba, T.. (2004). Germinated barley foodstuff prolongs remission in patients with ulcerative colitis. *International Journal of Molecular Medicine*, 13, 5, pp. (643-647), ISSN: 1107-3756.

Hanauer, S. B. (2004). Review article: aminosalicylates in inflammatory bowel disease. *Alimentary Pharmacology & Therapeutics*, 20 Suppl 4, pp. (60-65), ISSN: 0953-0673.

Hirsch, S., Schehlmann, V., Kolter, K., Bauer, K.H. (1995). Novel polymeric excipients for colon-targeting. *Macromolecular Symposia*. 99, 1, pp. (209-218), ISSN: 1157-1489.

Inan, M., Rasoulpour, R., Yin, L., Hubbard, A., Rosenberg, D., & Giardina, C. (2000). The luminal short-chain fatty acid butyrate modulates NF-κB activity in a human colonic epithelial cell line. *Gastroenterology*. 118, 4, pp. (724-734), ISSN: 0016-5085.

Jacobasch, G., Schmiedl, D., Kruschewski, M., & Schmehl, K. (1999). Dietary resistant starch and chronic inflammatory bowel diseases. *International Journal of Colorectal Disease*, 14, 4-5, pp. (201-211), ISSN: 0179-1958.

Jain, A., Gupta, Y., & Jain, S. K. (2007). Perspectives of biodegradable natural polysaccharides for site-specific drug delivery to the colon. *Journal of Pharmacy & Pharmaceutical Sciences : A Publication of the Canadian Society for Pharmaceutical Sciences*, 10, 1, pp. (86-128).

James, S. L., Muir, J. G., Curtis, S. L., & Gibson, P. R. (2003). Dietary fibre: a roughage guide. *Internal Medicine Journal*, 33, 7, pp. (291-296), ISSN: 1444-0903.

Jung, Y. J., Lee, J. S., Kim, H. H., Kim, Y. T., & Kim, Y. M. (1998). Synthesis and properties of dextran-5-aminosalicylic acid ester as a potential colon-specific prodrug of 5-aminosalicylic acid. *Archives of Pharmacal Research*, 21, 2, pp. (179-186), ISSN: 1976-3786.

Kanauchi, O., Serizawa, I., Araki, Y., Suzuki, A., Andoh, A., Fujiyama, Y., Mitsuyama, K., Takaki, K., Toyonaga, A., Sata, M., Bamba, T., Munakata, A., Ishiguro, Y. (2003). Germinated barley foodstuff, a prebiotic product, ameliorates inflammation of colitis through modulation of the enteric environment. *Journal of Gastroenterology*, 38, 2, pp. (134-41). doi: 10.1007/s005350300022.

Kanauchi, Osamu, Suga, T., Tochihara, M., Hibi, T., Naganuma, M., Homma, T., et al. (2002). Treatment of ulcerative colitis by feeding with germinated barley foodstuff: first report of a multicenter open control trial. *Journal of Gastroenterology*, 37 Suppl 1, pp. (67-72), ISSN: 0944-1174.

Le Blay, G., Michel, C., Blottière, H. M., & Cherbut, C. (1999). Prolonged intake of fructo-oligosaccharides induces a short-term elevation of lactic acid-producing bacteria and a persistent increase in cecal butyrate in rats. *The Journal of Nutrition*, 129, 12, pp. (2231-2235), ISSN: 0022-3166.

Liao, W., Cui, X. S., Jin, X. Y., & Floren, C. H. (1994). Lactulose–a potential drug for the treatment of inflammatory bowel disease. *Medical Hypotheses*, 43, 4, pp. (234–238), ISSN: 0306-9877.

Lin, S. Y., & Ayres, J. W. (1992). Calcium alginate beads as core carriers of 5-aminosalicylic acid. *Pharmaceutical Research*, 9, 9, pp. (1128-1131), ISSN: 0724-8741.

Lührs, H., Kudlich, T., Neumann, M., Schauber, J., Melcher, R., Gostner, A., Scheppach, W., Menzel, T. P.. (2002). Butyrate-enhanced TNFalpha-induced apoptosis is associated with inhibition of NF-kappaB. *Anticancer Research*, 22, 3, pp. (1561-1568). ISSN: 1043-4666.

Milojevic, S., Newton, J. M., Cummings, J. H., Gibson, G. R., Louise Botham, R., Ring, S. G., et al. (1996). Amylose as a coating for drug delivery to the colon: Preparation and in vitro evaluation using 5-aminosalicylic acid pellets. *Journal of Controlled Release*, 38, 1, pp. (75-84), ISSN: 0168-3659.

Mitsuyama, K, Saiki, T., Kanauchi, O, Iwanaga, T., Tomiyasu, N., Nishiyama, T., Tateishi, H., Shirachi, A., Ide, M., Suzuki, A., Noguchi, K., Ikeda, H., Toyonaga, A., & Sata, M. (1998). Treatment of ulcerative colitis with germinated barley foodstuff feeding: a pilot study. *Alimentary Pharmacology & Therapeutics*, 12, 12, pp. (1225-1230), ISSN: 0269-2813.

Moreau, N. M., Martin, L. J., Toquet, C. S., Laboisse, C. L., Nguyen, P. G., Siliart, B. S., Dumon, H. J., & Champ, M. J. (2007). Restoration of the integrity of rat caeco-colonic mucosa by resistant starch, but not by fructo-oligosaccharides, in dextran sulfate sodium-induced experimental colitis. *British Journal of Nutrition*, 90, 02, pp. (75-85), ISSN: 0007-1145.

Osterman, M. T., & Lichtenstein, G. R. (2009). Reformulation of an aminosalicylate: An example of the importance of pill burden on medical compliance rates. *Methods and Findings in Experimental and Clinical Pharmacology*, 31, 1, pp. (41–46), ISSN: 0379-0355.

Raghavan, C. V., Muthulingam, C., Jenita, J. A. J. L., & Ravi, T. K. (2002). An in vitro and in vivo investigation into the suitability of bacterially triggered delivery system for colon targeting. *Chemical & Pharmaceutical Bulletin*, 50, 7, pp. (892-895), ISSN: 0009-2363.

Rasmussen, S. N., Bondesen, S., Hvidberg, E. F., Hansen, S. H., Binder, V., Halskov, S., & Flachs, H. (1982). 5-aminosalicylic acid in a slow-release preparation: bioavailability, plasma level, and excretion in humans. *Gastroenterology*, 83, 5, pp. (1062-1070), ISSN: 0016-5085.

Rodriguez-Cabezas, M. E., Galvez, J., Lorente, M. D., Concha, A., Azzouz, S., Camuesco, D., Azzouz, S., Osuna, A., Redondo, L, & Zarzuelo, A. (2002). Biochemical and Molecular Actions of Nutrients Dietary Fiber Down-Regulates Colonic Tumor Necrosis Factor and Nitric Oxide Production in Trinitrobenzenesulfonic Acid-Induced Colitic Rats. *Journal of Nutrition*, 132, 11, pp. (3263-3271), ISSN: 0022-3166.

Rose, D. J., & Hamaker, B. R. (2011). Chapter 8 Overview of Dietary Fiber and its Influence on Gastrointestinal Health, In: *Nondigestible Carbohydrates and Digestive Health*, Paeschke, T.M. and Aimutis, W.R., pp. (185-221), Wiley-Blackwell, ISBN: 978-0-8138-1762-0.

Rumi, G., Tsubouchi, R., Okayama, M., Kato, S., Mózsik, G., & Takeuchi, Koji. (2004). Protective effect of lactulose on dextran sulfate sodium-induced colonic inflammation in rats. *Digestive Diseases and Sciences*, 49, 9, pp. (1466-1472), ISSN: 0163-2116.

Sandborn, W.J. (2006). New Advances in 5-ASA Therapy for Ulcerative Colitis, In: *Medscape Gastroenterology*, June 22, 2011, Available from: <http://www.medscape.org/viewarticle/553568>.

Sandborn, W.J. (2006). Treatment of ulcerative colitis with oral mesalamine: Advances in drug formulation, efficacy expectations and dose response, compliance, and chemoprevention. *Reviews in Gastroenterological Disorders*, 6, 2, pp. (97-105), ISSN: 1533-001X.

Sartor, R. B. (2006). Mechanisms of disease: pathogenesis of Crohn's disease and ulcerative colitis. *Nature clinical practice. Gastroenterology & Hepatology*, 3, 7, pp. (390-407). doi: 10.1038/ncpgasthep0528.

Selby, W. S., Barr, G. D., Ireland, A., Mason, C. H., Jewell, D. P., & Selby, S. (2011). Olsalazine In Active Ulcerative Colitis. *British Medical Journal*, 291, 6506, pp. (1373-1375), ISSN: 0007-1447.

Thimma, R.T. & Tammishetti, S. (2001). Barium chloride crosslinked carboxymethyl guar gum beads for gastrointestinal drug delivery, *Journal of Applied Polymer Science*, 82, 12, pp. (3084-3090), ISSN: 0021-8995.

Van den Mooter, G., Vervoort, L., & Kinget, R. (2003). Characterization of methacrylated inulin hydrogels designed for colon targeting: in vitro release of BSA. *Pharmaceutical Research*, 20, 2, pp. (303-307), ISSN: 0724-8741.

Videla, S., Vilaseca, J., & Antolín, M. (2001). Dietary inulin improves distal colitis induced by dextran sodium sulfate in the rat. *The American Journal of Gastroenterology*, 96, 5, pp. (1486-1493), ISSN: 0002-9270.

Vilivalam, V., Illum, I., & Iqbal, I. (2000). Starch capsules: an alternative system for oral drug delivery. *Pharmaceutical Science & Technology Today*, 3, 2, pp. (64-69), ISSN: 1461-5347.

Wong, T. W., Colombo, G., & Sonvico, F. (2011). Pectin matrix as oral drug delivery vehicle for colon cancer treatment. *AAPS PharmSciTech*, 12, 1, pp. (201-214), ISSN: 1530-9932.

Zou, M., Okamoto, H., Cheng, G., Hao, X., Sun, J., Cui, F., & Danjo, K. (2005). Synthesis and properties of polysaccharide prodrugs of 5-aminosalicylic acid as potential colon-specific delivery systems. *European Journal of Pharmaceutics and Biopharmaceutics : Official Journal of Arbeitsgemeinschaft für Pharmazeutische Verfahrenstechnik e.V*, 59, 1, pp. (155-160), ISSN: 0939-6411.

7

Food and Intestinal Microorganisms: Factors in Pathogenesis, Prevention and Therapy of Ulcerative Colitis

Rok Orel and Darja Urlep
University Medical Centre Ljubljana, Children's Hospital, Department of Gastroenterology, Hepatology and Nutrition
Slovenia

1. Introduction

Ulcerative colitis (UC) is a chronic and relapsing inflammatory disease of the large bowel characterized by dysregulation of the immune mucosal response, an imbalance in the synthesis and release of cytokines, and an unresolved inflammatory process associated with mucosal damage (Schirbel & Fiocchi, 2010).

Although the exact mechanisms of the development of UC have not been established yet, it is known that both genetic predisposition and environmental factors are playing important roles. There is the strong evidence that environmental factors are involved in the pathogenesis of UC. The incidence of UC has increased dramatically between 1940s and the 1980s. More recent data show that, in several developed countries, UC incidence decreases in the last years (Binder, 2004). On the other hand, at the same time, the incidence of UC increased in countries where it formally was low (e.g. developing countries and developed countries in Asia, such as Japan and Korea). It is believed that factors associated with 'Westernization' may be conditioning the expression of UC. The increased incidence of UC among migrants from the low-incidence to high-incidence areas within the same or next generation confirms a strong environmental influence (Bernstein & Shanahan, 2008).

Another evidence for the role of environmental factors in UC comes from twin studies: disease concordance in monozygotic twins is only 19% in UC, as opposed to 50% in Crohn's disease (CD). This observation suggests that the environmental influence is stronger in UC than in CD (Halfvarson et al., 2003).

In the last decades several environmental factors, and especially the diet and the changes of the gut microbiota have been studied to improve our understanding of increased incidence of inflammatory bowel disease (IBD) in the last years and also to elucidate the pathogenesis of the disease.

2. Diet as a risk factor for the development of ulcerative colitis

The evidence about the role of dietary factors in UC etiology is relatively scarce. However, over the past few decades, several studies have highlighted the potential association between diet and the risk of UC.

Some studies have shown that breastfeeding reduces the risk of development of UC (Corrao et al., 1998) and CD (Koletzko et al., 1989). There are also some studies which could not confirm the positive association between breastfeeding and subsequent development of UC (Koletzko et al., 1989). In 2004, a systematic review and meta-analysis reported a significant protective effect of breastfeeding against both CD and UC (Klement et al., 2004). The role of breastfeeding in the development of childhood onset IBD (<16 years of age) was assessed in the meta-analysis by Barclay et al. Breast milk exposure had a significant protective effect (OR, 0.69; 95% CI, 0.51-0.94; P=0.02) in a developing childhood onset IBD (Barclay et al., 2009). However, the quality of existing data from the included studies was poor, therefore, the role of breastfeeding as a protective factor in developing IBD needs to be investigated in well-designed prospective studies.

In the developed countries with high incidence of IBD, »western lifestyle« includes new feeding habits in which the consumption of high quantities of refined sugar, fat, red meat and the low consumption of dietary fiber, fruit and vegetables take precedence.

In patients with IBD, many studies on sucrose consumption have been conducted since Martini et al. reported in 1976 that patients with CD consumed an excess amount of sugar- and sugar-containing products (Martini et al., 1976). Some other studies have confirmed that ingestion of large amount of refined sugars may be a possible risk factor in the development of IBD (Persson et al., 1992; Reif et al., 1997). The proposed mechanism is the influence of sugars on the composition of intestinal microbiota. In a case control study by Russel et al. the consumption of cola drinks and chocolate consumption were positively associated with developing ulcerative colitis (Russel et al., 1998). A multicenter Japanese study showed that a higher consumption of sweets was positively associated with UC risk and that the intake of vitamin C was negatively related to UC risk (Sakamoto et al., 2005). However, some other studies on the role of refined sugars in the etiology of UC did not confirm the association between the intake of higher amount of refined sugars and development of UC. Therefore, larger prospective studies are needed to elucidate the role of refined sugars in the etiology of IBD.

Several studies reported that the high intake of fats was associated with an increased risk of UC. In a study by Geerling et al. high intakes of monounsaturated and polyunsaturated fat were associated with an increased risk to develop UC (Geerling et al., 2000).

The large European Prospective Investigation into Cancer and Nutrition (EPIC) study from over 200,000 subjects across five European countries assessed dietary data in subjects who were diagnosed with UC compared to control subjects. The study showed a significant positive correlation between the dietary content of linoleic acid (omega-6-fatty acid) and increased incidence of UC, and a negative association with intake of docosahexaenoic acid (omega-3-fatty acid) (Tjonneland et al., 2009).

In a recent British study investigating the total dietary intake of omega-3 polyunsaturated fatty acids (PUFAs) and the specific omega-3 PUFAs, eicosapentaenoic acid (EPA) and docosahexaenoic acid (DHA) on the risk of developing incident UC, the total dietary omega-3 PUFAs, EPA, and DHA were associated with protection from UC in a large cohort of subjects aged over 45 years. Authors concluded that increasing the population's intake of omega-3 PUFAs from oily fish may help prevent UC (John et al., 2010).

Hou et al. performed a systematic review of possible association between pre-diagnosis dietary intake and risk of developing IBD and have identified 19 studies (18 case-control and one cohort) with 2,609 IBD patients (1,269 CD and 1,340 UC and over 4,000 controls). Studies reported that high intakes of total fats, PUFAs, omega-6 PUFAs, and meat were consistently associated with increased risk of developing UC as well as CD. High vegetable intake was associated with decreased risk of developing UC, whereas fiber and fruit intake was associated with reduced risk of CD (Hou et al., 2011). However, this systematic review is affected by the limitations of the individual studies and potential publication bias against negative studies. Furthermore, studies are heterogeneous in study design, nutrient cut-offs and study populations. The retrospective nature of the majority of studies may have resulted in recall bias involving IBD cases. Therefore, further prospective studies will be needed to elucidate the association between dietary factors and the risk of UC as well as CD.

3. The role of nutrition in the therapy of ulcerative colitis

Inflammatory bowel disease is frequently associated with nutritional deficiencies in calories, macro- and micro-nutrients. Malnutrition is common in active CD, however, nutritional deficiencies can develop fast also in UC patients, especially during periods of active disease. The pattern and severity of nutritional deficiencies depends on the extent, activity and duration of the inflammation (Lucendo & De Rezende, 2009). Nutritional deficiencies are especially common in both pediatric CD and UC, therefore, the nutritional support is especially important in childhood IBD. Providing macronutrients can improve growth. Identifying and correcting micronutrient deficiencies can improve comorbid conditions like osteopenia and anemia (Mallon & Suskind, 2010). Malnutrition and specific deficits, e.g. of iron, zinc, selenium, water and lipid soluble vitamins, are a consequence of several mechanisms: apetite loss, increased energy consumption, malabsorption, intestinal losses, changes in metabolism due to systemic inflammatory cytokine effects and drug therapy. Therefore, the main purpose of nutritional treatment of IBD is to provide adequate intake of all macro- and micronutrients to compensate for existing deficiencies and to cope with increased demands. Specialized nutritional formulas for IBD patients are produced that ensure adequate and complete intake of all necessary nutrients. Exclusive enteral nutrition (EN) is an established primary therapy for pediatric CD and allows the inflammatory activity to be controlled and kept in remission, however enteral nutrition does not have a primary role in the therapy of ulcerative colitis (Otley et al., 2010).

Nutritional support in IBD is frequently used to treat malnutrition, however there is also an attempt to modulate intestinal inflammation. Nutrients may be involved in the modulation of the immune response as components of cell membranes, they can also mediate the expression of proteins involved in the immune response, especially the cytokines and adhesion molecules. Immunologic mechanisms have been also postulated to link food antigens and the development of intestinal inflammation (Torres & Ríos, 2008).

The emerging concepts of nutrition-gene interaction gave birth to unique scientific fields, nutrigenetics and nutrigenomics. These studies provide information about the genetic variability that induces an individual's response to nutrition and changes in gene expression that develop as a result of food-gene interaction. In IBD, the role of diet in the regulation of the immune response to gut microbiota is the subject of current intensive evaluation. These approaches may lead clinicians to derive a personalized nutritional prescription based on individual genetic variations and may result in a significant impact on IBD treatment (Ferguson, 2010).

Intestinal immune responses could be modulated by supplementation with specific immunomodulatory amino acids. Experimental studies evaluating glutamine, the preferential substrate for enterocytes, are promising. The role of arginine, involved in nitric oxide and polyamines synthesis, still remains debated. However, the effects of these amino acids and other candidates like glycine, cysteine, histidine, or taurine should be evaluated in the future (Coëffier et al., 2010).

3.1 The role of fats in ulcerative colitis

Many studies have confirmed the important role of lipids in the diet to regulate inflammatory processes in different diseases, as they are the fundamental component of cell membranes, including those of lymphocytes and other immune cells, which orchestrate immune system responses (Ioannidis et al., 2011). Some studies have shown that high-fat diets have been associated with an imbalance between effector T cells and regulatory T cells and therefore with increased risk for UC what was confirmed in mouse models of experimental colitis. Mice receiving the high-fat diet were more susceptible to experimental-induced colitis compared to mice fed a normal diet (Jeffery et al., 1997).

The observation that the Eskimos in Greenland, consumers of large quantities of omega-3 PUFAs deriving from fish oils, had a low prevalence of IBD, led to the study of the anti-inflammatory properties of omega-3 PUFAs in comparison with pro-inflammatory omega-6 PUFAs (Bang et al., 1980).

Polyunsaturated fatty acids are involved in the immune response as they are precursors of the eicosanoids. Omega-3 PUFAs are considered to have a beneficial effect in the management of IBD by repressing cytokine production and modulating the production of eicosanoids. Omega-3 PUFAs compete with omega-6 PUFAs in the substrate pool of the lipooxygenase pathway, thus reducing the production of inflammatory eicosanoids like leukotriene B_4 (LTB_4) and thromboxane A_2. They cause a shift from LTB_4 to LTB_5 production which is less bioactive (Calder, 2009).

All the mechanisms through which the omega-3 PUFAs perform their immunomodulating action still remain unclear. Changing the fatty acid composition of immune cells also affects T cell reactivity and antigen presentation. Fatty acids can also influence cytokine (TNF-alfa, IL-1) production. To a certain extent this action may be due to the altered profile of regulatory eicosanoids, but it seems likely that eicosanoid-independent actions are a more important mechanisms. Indeed, effects on transcription factors that regulate inflammatory gene expression (e.g. nuclear factor kappaB) seem to be important (Galli & Calder, 2009). Recently, Vieira de Barros et al. demonstrated that the soybean (source of omega-6 PUFAs) and fish oil (source of omega-3 PUFAs) mixture, more than fish oil alone, increased IL-10/IL-4 ratio (anti-inflammatory/pro-inflammatory) in experimental dextran sodium sulphate-induced colitis rats to levels closer to the control group of non-colitis rats (Vieira de Barros et al., 2011). This finding shows that a balanced omega-3/omega-6 diet may be a key factor which could exert beneficial effects in UC. Indeed, many current »Western diets« provide a high omega-6/omega-3 ratio of over 15:1 and it is recommended that human diet should return to a more balanced omega-6/omega-3 ratio of around 1:4 or less.

Dietary fatty acids are also important risk factors in carcinogenesis due to their lipid peroxidation products. The omega-6 PUFAs have been considered to increase lipid peroxidation via cyclooxygenases, while omega-3 PUFAs exerts a chemopreventive role by suppressing the formation of lipid peroxidation products derived from arachidonic acid oxidation through competitive inhibition of desaturases (Rose & Connolly, 1999). It is well known that patients with UC have increased risk of developing colorectal cancer (CRC), therefore, the consumption of appropriate amount of omega-3 PUFAs may be beneficial in the prevention of CRC.

Although fish oil supplementation in patients with IBD results in omega-3 PUFAs incorporation into gut mucosal tissue and modification of inflammatory mediator profiles, the evidence of clinical benefits of omega-3 PUFAs is conflicting. Some studies have demonstrated the efficacy of fish oil and omega-3 PUFAs in the management of UC (Hawthorne et al., 1992; Stenson et al., 1992), however, a meta-analysis performed by Turner et al. in 2007 found no evidence that supports the use of omega-3 PUFAs (fish oil) for maintenance of remission in UC (Turner et al., 2007).

In a recent systematic review and meta-analysis of the efficacy and safety of omega-3 PUFAs (and fish oil) for maintaining remission in CD and UC, the same authors came to the same conclusion. Nine studies were eligible for inclusion; six studies of 1039 CD patients and three studies of 138 UC patients. For UC, there was no difference in the relapse rate between the omega-3 and control groups (RR 1.02; 95% CI: 0.51-2.03). Additionally, the analysis showed a higher rate of diarrhea and symptoms of the upper gastrointestinal tract in the omega-3 treatment group. The authors concluded that there were insufficient data to recommend the use of omega 3 PUFAs for maintenance of remission in CD and UC (Turner et al., 2011).

3.2 The role of short-chain fatty acids in ulcerative colitis

The multiple beneficial effects on human health of the short-chain fatty acids (SCFA) are well documented. SCFAs are organic acids produced by intestinal microbial fermentation of mainly undigested dietary carbohydrates, specifically resistant starches and dietary fiber, but also in a minor part by dietary and endogenous proteins. SCFAs are essentially produced in the colon. The ratio of SCFA concentrations in the colonic lumen is about 60% acetate, 25% propionate, and 15% butyrate. As a result of increasing concentrations of acidic fermentation products, the luminal pH in the proximal colon is lower. The ability to produce butyrate is widely distributed among the Gram-positive anaerobic bacteria that inhabit the human colon. Numerically, two of the most important groups of butyrate producers appear to be *Faecalibacterium prausnitzii,* which belongs to the *Clostridium leptum* (or clostridial cluster IV) cluster, and *Eubacterium rectale/Roseburia spp.,* which belong to the *Clostridium coccoides* (or clostridial cluster XIVa) cluster of firmicute bacteria (Canani et al., 2011).

Short-chain fatty acids and, especially, butyrate play a very important role in the biology of the large bowel epithelium, representing the primary energy source of the large bowel cell. They have been proposed to play a key role in the maintenance of colonic homeostasis. Deficiency of SCFA in the intestinal lumen is related with epithelium atrophy and inflammation. Butyrate has a role as an anti-inflammatory agent, primarily via inhibition of nuclear factor κB (NF-κB) activation in human colonic epithelial cells. NF-κB regulates many cellular genes involved in early immune inflammatory responses, including IL-1b, TNF-α, IL-2, IL-6, IL-8, IL-12, intercellular adhesion molecule-1 (ICAM-1), T cell receptor-α (TCR-α), and MHC class II molecules. It is well known that the activity of NF-κB is dysregulated in inflammatory bowel diseases (Guilloteau et al., 2011).

Short-chain fatty acids have potent effects on a variety of colonic mucosal functions such as inhibition of carcinogenesis and reinforcing various components of the colonic defence barrier and decreasing oxidative stress. Butyrat is also a potential promoter of the proliferation and differentiation of large intestine epithelial cells and reduces the paracellular permeability, possibly due to the promotion of intestinal cell differentiation. At the intestinal level, butyrate plays a regulatory role on the transepithelial fluid transport and modulates visceral sensitivity and intestinal motility. In vivo studies have shown that butyrate has the pro-absorptive and anti-secretory effect in the distal colon. The mechanisms of action of butyrate are different; many of these are related to its potent regulatory effects on gene expression (Kovarik et al., 2011).

Several studies have reported that butyrate metabolism is impaired in intestinal mucosa of patients with IBD (Hamer et al., 2008). In UC butyrate oxidation has been shown to be disturbed, but it remains unclear whether this is a primary defect (De Preter et al., 2009). Recently some in vivo studies using biopsy specimens of inflamed mucosa have shown the impaired anti-inflammatory efficacy of n-butyrate in patients with IBD. There is a reduction of butyrate uptake by the inflamed mucosa. The concomitant induction of the glucose transporter GLUT1 suggests that inflammation could induce a metabolic switch from butyrate to glucose oxidation. Butyrate transport deficiency is expected to have clinical consequences. Particularly, the reduction of the intracellular availability of butyrate in colonocytes may decrease its protective effects toward cancer in IBD patients (Canani et al., 2011).

Considering the various beneficial effects of butyrate, it is expected that the administration of butyrate could alleviate the symptoms associated with intestinal inflammation in IBD. The addition of butyrat to standard mesalazine treatment in patients with UC has led to marked improvement of symptoms and endoscopic appearance of mucosa, thus proving effective in reducing disease activity (Assisi et al., 2008). In an Italian double blind, placebo-controlled multicenter trial, 51 patients with active distal UC were treated with rectal enemas containing either 5-aminosalicylic acid (5-ASA) or 5-ASA plus sodium butyrate (80 mmol/L, twice a day). The combined treatment with topical 5-ASA plus sodium butyrate significantly improved the disease activity score more than 5-ASA alone (Vernia et al., 2003). In a study by Hallert et al. an addition of 60 g oat bran (corresponding to 20 g dietary fiber) to the daily diet of patients with quiescent UC resulted in a significant increase of fecal butyrate concentration and in a significant improvement of abdominal symptoms (Hallert et al., 2003). On the other hand, in a recent study by Hamer et al. only minor effects on inflammatory and oxidative stress parameters were observed in UC patients in remission who were treated with rectal butyrate enemas (Hamer et al., 2010).

Although most studies point towards beneficial effects of butyrate, more human in vivo studies are needed to contribute to our current understanding of butyrate-mediated effects on colonic function and its clinical efficacy in reducing inflammation in UC.

4. The role of microbiota in the pathogenesis of ulcerative colitis

Most recent theories regard IBD as a consequence of abnormal mucosal immune response to antigens of gut bacterial microbiota in genetically susceptible individuals.

Previous studies have focused on identifying specific pathogenic microorganisms responsible for IBD. However, further studies have not confirmed the role of specific infectious agents in the pathogenesis of IBD. Moreover, there is growing evidence that the normal bacterial microbiota can trigger harmful immune reactions in susceptible hosts. The most convincing evidence supporting the role of enteric microbiota in the pathogenesis of IBD comes from animal studies. Animals with genetically engineered dysregulation of the immune response developed spontaneous colitis, when they were growing in the normal conditions resembling IBD in humans. However, they did not develop intestinal inflammation when they were growing in a germ free environment indicating that bacterial exposure and colonization of the gut are essential for the development of colitis (Sellon et al., 1998). Interleukin-10 (IL-10) deficient mice displayed a significantly higher number of mucosal adherent bacteria and lower level of protective bacteria like *Lactobacillus* compared to healthy mice. The proportion of mucosal adherent bacteria and the development of colitis were significantly decreased by nutritional supplementation of lactose or enema delivery of *Lactobacillus reuteri* (Madsen et al., 1999). Similarly, *Lactobacillus plantarum* attenuated established colonic inflammation in IL-10 deficient mice as was manifested by decreased histological colitis score and mucosal cytokines IL-12, interferon gamma (IFN-gamma) and immunoglobulin G2a level (Schultz et al., 2002).

Several studies in humans have observed the role of gut microbiota in the pathogenesis of IBD. The inflammation of gut mucosa and consequent lesions occur predominantly in the areas with the highest bacterial counts like terminal ileum and colon (Sartor, 1997). Rutgeerts et al. reported that the recurrence of mucosal inflammation in the neoterminal ileum after curative ileal resection in patients with IBD was dependent on the fecal stream. The relapse of the inflammation occurred after the restoration of the fecal stream (Rutgeerts et al., 1991). In a study by D'Haens et al. early IBD lesions were induced in susceptible individuals by the direct installation of fecal material into non-inflamed loops of the intestine (D'Haens et al., (1998).

Human studies have repeatedly shown that microbiota of patients with IBD differs from that of controls and is unstable, both in the intestinal lumen and on the surface of the mucosa (Chassaing et al., 2011). A single pathogen has not been identified, but potentially pro-inflammatory micro-organisms have been found in the mucosal samples from IBD patients more often than from healthy controls. Shifts in the composition of resident bacteria in CD and UC patients have been postulated to drive the chronic inflammation seen in both diseases (the »dysbiosis hypothesis«) (Marteau, 2009).

The gut microbiota composition in IBD shows a decreased prevalence of dominant members of the human commensal microbiota (*Bifidobacterium* and *Lactobacillus* species, *Clostridium* IXa and IV groups) and a concomitant increase in detrimental bacteria (sulphate-reducing bacteria, adherent/invasive *Escherichia coli*) (Fava& Danese, 2011).

Considering the important role of intestinal microbiota in the development and maintenance of intestinal inflammation in IBD, many efforts have been made to find ways to influence on bacterial composition in a way to decrease inflammation and prevent exacerbations. With this intention, pre- and probiotis are increasingly used (Sartor, 2004).

5. The role of prebiotics in ulcerative colitis

Prebiotics are defined as nondigestible food ingredients that beneficially affect the host by selectively stimulating the growth or activity of one or a limited number of bacterial species already resident in the colon. Therefore, the rationale behind prebiotic use is to increase the populations of certain endogenic beneficial bacteria such as *Lactobacillus* and *Bifidobacterium*. This change may act beneficially by causing luminal production of SCFA, which induce acidic environment, by preventing of pathogenic bacteria adherence and by production of anti-bacterial substances (Roberfroid et al., 2010).

Prebiotics are usually in the form of oligosaccharides, which may occur naturally but can also be added as dietary supplements to foods, beverages, and infant formula. Prebiotic oligosaccharides often contain fructose chains with a terminal glucose and typically consist of 10 or fewer sugar molecules. Examples of prebiotic oligosaccharides include fructooligosaccharides (FOS), galactooligosaccharides (GOS) and inulin. Inulin and FOS are composed of multiple saccharide units, which are indigestible by the human enzymes. They stimulate the growth of lactic acid bacteria and the generation of SCFA (Thomas & Greer, 2010).

Although several prebiotic compounds possess promising properties to have beneficial effect in IBD, only few of them have been clinically tested.

In dextran sodium sulphate (DSS) - induced colitis of an animal model, inulin attenuated gut inflammation (Videla et al., 2001). Similarly, FOS were shown to decrease the severity of damage of the intestinal mucosa in the experimental model of rat colitis (Cherbut et al., (2003). Psyllium, also called Ispaghula husk or Plantago ovata, is a water soluble dietary fiber. Hallert et al. reported that Ispaghula husk had significantly attenuated symptoms in patients with UC (Hallert et al., 1991) and Spanish Group for the Study of Crohn's Disease and Ulcerative Colitis (GETECCU) found it as efficient as sulfasalazine in maintaining remission in UC (Fernandez-Banares et al., 1999).

Germinated barley foodstuff (GBF) is derived from aleurone layer and scutellum fractions of germinated barley and consists mainly of dietary fiber and glutamine-rich protein. It induces intestinal microflora to produce SCFA (Kanauchi et al., 1999). Treatment of rat experimental colitis with GBF led to improvement of the clinical and pathological signs of colitis and decreased serum cytokine production (Kanauchi et al., 2003). The same Japanese group reported the efficacy of GBF in some studies in patients with active UC and UC in remission (Kanauchi et al., 2003; Hanai et al., 2004). According to these results, GBF has been registered as a special foodstuff for UC by Japan's Ministry of Health, Labor and Welfare.

Given the important influences on intestinal microbiota and immune functions, prebiotics are considered as a promising tool in the management and prevention of IBD in the future. However, larger and well-designed clinical studies are necessary to elucidate the efficacy of prebiotics in patients with UC.

6. The role of probiotics in ulcerative colitis

Probiotics are defined as live microorganisms which, when administered in adequate amounts, confer a health benefit on the host. Multiple mechanisms of action have been suggested to explain the effect of probiotics in IBD. These mechanisms include suppression of growth, epithelial binding and invasion by pathogenic bacteria, production of antimicrobial substances, improved epithelial barrier function, and immunoregulation (Collado et al., 2009).

A large body of data is showing a great potential of probiotic use in the treatment of IBD patients. The effects of probiotics are both strain- and dose - dependent. For example, the probiotic *Lactobacillus rhamnosus* GG (LGG) attenuated the TNF-alfa induced IL-8 production at doses $10^{6\text{-}8}$ by the Caco-2 intestinal cell line, but on the contrary, at higher doses the level of IL-8 was increased by the same probiotic (Zhang et al., 2005). This finding indicates that the determination of the correct dose of a probiotic is of crucial importance for the appropriate treatment efficacy. The same study demonstrated also that heat-killed LGG was also able to decrease IL-8 production. This observation denied the paradigm that viability of probiotics is essential for their efficacy. Similarly, bacterial DNA from VSL#3, a high dose mixture of three strains of *Bifidobacteria,* four strains of *Lactobacilli,* and one strain of *Streptococcus salivarius* ssp. *thermophilus,* was able to decrease IL-8 secretion, delay NF-κB activation and stabilize IkappaB levels (Jijon et al., 2004). However, in another study using *Lactobacillus reuteri* on HT-29 and T84 cells only live but not deactivated bacteria reduced TNF-alfa induced IL-8 production and induced production of anti-inflammatory factors (Ma et al., 2004).

The most convincing evidence of the probiotic efficacy and mechanisms of action comes from animal studies. These experiments clearly demonstrated that the effect of probiotic treatment depends both on the probiotic strain and the type of experimental inflammation. Not only live bacteria, but also soluble bacterial antigens extracted from different probiotic strains showed the ability to reduce the inflammation (Evaschuk et al., 2006). Therefore, viability of probiotic bacteria was not proven to be a prerequisite for their effect.

Author (year)	Probiotic	Treatment duration	N.(probiotic /control group)	Outcome N (probiotic/control group)
Kruis et al., 1997	*E. coli* Nissle 1917	12 wk	50/53	Maintenance of remission 42/51
Rembacken et al., 1999	*E. coli* Nissle 1917	12 mo	57/59	Induction of remission 39/44 Maintenance of remission 31/27
Ishikawa et al., 2003	Bifidobacteria-fermented milk (BFM)	12 mo	11/10	Maintenance of remission 8/1
Kruis et al., 2004	*E. coli* Nissle 1917	12 mo	162/165	Maintenance of remission 98/104
Cui et al., 2004	*Bifidobacteria* (3 strains)	8 wk	15/15	Maintenance of remission 12/1
Kato et al., 2004	*B. breve* strain Yakult, *B. bifidum* strain Yakult, *Lactobacillus Acidophilus*	12 wk	10/10	Induction of remission 4/3
Tursi et al., 2004	VSL#3	8 wk	30/30/30	Maintenance of remission 24/21/16
Furrie et al., 2005	*Bifidobacterium longum* +prebiotics	4 wk	9/9	Induction of remission 5/3
Sood et al., 2009	VSL#3	12 wk	77/70	Induction of remission 33/11
Miele et al., 2009	VSL#3	12 mo	14/15	Induction of remission 13/4 Maintenance of remission 11/4

Table 1. Randomized, controlled trials examining the effects of probiotics in inducing and/or maintaining remission in patients with ulcerative colitis

In the last years, many studies on the role of probiotics in UC have been published, however, many of them are small and methodologically weak. In the table 1 only randomized controlled clinical trials (RCT) addressing the role of probiotics in inducing and/or maintaining remission in patients with UC, published in the last years, are shown.

Rembacken et al. reported that probiotics (*E. coli* Nissle 1917) with steroids had similar efficacy compared to mesalazine with steroids in achieving remission, however, the relapse rate was slightly higher in the mesalazine group compared to probiotic group (73% vs. 67%, $P < 0.05$) (Rembacken et al., 1999). In 2004, Kato utilized a yogurt with *Bifidobacterium breve* strain Yakult, *B. bifidum* strain Yakult and a *L. acidophilus* strain, in addition to therapy with 5-ASA, in 20 patients with mild-to-moderate UC, and showed that this treatment was superior to conventional treatment alone in inducing remission as judged by clinical and endoscopic parameters (Kato et al., 2004). Tursi et al. used the probiotic mixture VSL#3 in 90 adults with mild-to-moderate active UC. In the probiotic group patients were treated with balsalazide and probiotic VSL#3. The first placebo group was treated with balsalazide alone and the second placebo group with mesalazine alone. Although they did not find the statistical significant difference in the proportion of patients of all three groups in achieving remission, the mean time to remission was significantly shorter in the probiotic group (4 vs 7 days, $P < 0.01$) (Tursi et al., 2004).

In a study by Kruis et al. there was no difference between the probiotic drug E coli Nissle 1917 and the standard therapy with mesalazine in maintaining remission in patients with ulcerative colitis (Kruis et al., 2004). In 2005, Furrie et al. reported results in 18 patients with active UC treated with a synbiotic preparation: a combination of a probiotic (*B. longum*) and a prebiotic (»Synergy 1«, an inulin-oligofructose polymer). The patients on the synbiotic appeared to have achieved clinical and endoscopic remission sooner, although the difference was only borderline significant ($p=0.06$) (Furrie et al., 2005). Miele et al. conducted the only published pediatric RCT on probiotics. In the study, children with a newly diagnosed mild or moderate UC were randomly assigned to receive either prednisone and mesalazine plus placebo, or prednisone and mesalazine plus VSL#3. At the end of induction therapy after 4 weeks, significantly more patients were in full remission if on VSL#3. In addition, colonoscopic and pathological scores assessed at 6 and 12 months were also significantly better in children on VSL#3. The percentage of patients without relapse at 1 year (80 vs 30%) was significantly better for the patients on the probiotic (Miele et al., 2009). A recent meta-analysis by Li-Xuan Sang et al. showed that using probiotics provided no additional benefit in inducing remission of ulcerative colitis. On the other hand, the probiotics auxiliary therapy was much better than non-probiotics therapy for maintenance treatment of UC (Li-Xuan et al., 2010). Based on the clinical trial evidence, available to date, *E. coli* Nissle and VSL#3 appear to be most effective in the management of UC. Therapy with *E. coli* Nissle 1917 for maintenance of remission of UC is now recommended in some European guidelines on the treatment of UC (Stange et al., 2008). Pouchitis, chronic inflammation of ileal pouch created after proctocolectomy, may occur in approximately 30% of patients and is usually treated by antibiotics. However, in the last decade, the clinical efficacy of probiotic use in the maintaining of remission and the prevention of pouchitis was observed. Gionchetti et al. compared the efficacy of VSL#3 with placebo in maintenance of remission of pouchitis. The patients in the probiotic group relapsed in 15% when compared with 100% in the placebo group (Gionchetti et al., 2000). These results were replicated by Mimura et al. They found that the relapse rate after 12 months from the beginning of the therapy was 15% for VSL#3 group versus 94% for the placebo group (Mimura et al., 2004). In another study by Gionchetti et al. the efficacy of probiotic VSL#3 in the prevention of pouchitis after colectomy and pouch surgery was confirmed. During the first year after the operation, 10% of the patients on probiotic VSL#3 and 40% of the patients on placebo developed pouchitis (Gionchetti et al., 2003). In contrast to probiotic VSL#3, the study with *Lactobacillus rhamnosus* GG observed alterations in intestinal microbiota but no other effects on clinical parameters (Kuisma et al., 2003). In a recent meta-analysis a search for randomized controlled trials (RCTs) of treatment and prevention of pouchitis from 1966 to October 2009 was performed. The primary objective was to determine the efficacy of medical therapies for pouchitis (including antibiotic, probiotic, and other agents) as substantiated by data from RCTs. For acute pouchitis, ciprofloxacin was more effective than metronidazole, while budesonide enemas and metronidazole were similarly effective. For chronic pouchitis, VSL#3 was more effective than placebo. For the prevention of pouchitis, VSL#3 was also more effective than placebo (Holubar et al., 2010). This meta-analysis confirmed the role of probiotic use for the treatment of chronic pouchitis and especially in prevention of pouchitis after ileal pouch-anal anastomosis.

7. Conclusion

The incidence of IBD in developed countries has increased over the last decades and is still increasing. The increase in the incidence cannot be explained only by the genetic background. Therefore, it is clear that the environmental factors play an important role. Several studies have been performed to clarify the role of nutritional factors in the development of UC and CD. There is some data showing that high intake of refined sugars, animal fat, red meat, omega-6 PUFAs and lower intake of omega-3 PUFAs may contribute to the increasing incidence of UC in the developed countries. Omega-3 PUFAs have been shown to have a beneficial effect in reducing gut mucosal inflammation, however, further studies have to be conducted to elucidate their exact role in the therapy of UC. Considering the important role of gut microbiota in the pathogenesis of UC, many efforts have already been made to change its composition in a way to decrease the inflammation and prevent exacerbations. With this intention, pre- and probiotics are being increasingly investigated. Clinical use of probiotics to date has been proved effective in the therapy of pouchitis and maintenance of remission in ulcerative colitis.

8. References

Assisi, RF, et al. (2008). Combined butyric acid/mesalazine treatment in ulcerative colitis with mild-moderate activity. Results of a multicentre pilot study. *Minerva gastroenterologica e dietologica*, Vol. 54, No. 3, (Sep 2008), pp. (231-238), ISSN 1121-421X

Bang, HO, et al. (1980). The composition of the Eskimo food in north western Greenland. *The American Journal of Clinical Nutrition*, Vol. 33, No. 12, (Dec 1980), pp. (2657-2661), ISSN 0002-9165

Barclay, AR, et al. (2009). Systematic review: the role of breastfeeding in the development of pediatric inflammatory bowel disease, *Journal of Pediatrics*, Vol. 155, No. 36792, (Sept 2009), pp. (421-426), ISSN 1309-1247

Bernstein, CN, & Shanahan, F. (2008). Disorders of a modern lifestyle: reconciling the epidemiology of inflammatory bowel disease, *Gut*, Vol. 57, No. 9 (May 2008), pp. (1185-1191), ISSN 0017-5749

Binder, V. (2004). Epidemiology of IBD during the twentieth century: an integrated view. *Best Practice & Research Clinical Gastroenterology*, Vol. 18, No. 3, (Jun 2004), pp. (463-79), ISSN 1521-6918

Calder, PC. (2009). Polyunsaturated fatty acids and inflammatory processes: New twists in an old tale. *Biochimie*, Vol. 91, No. 6, (Jun 2009), pp. (791-795), ISSN 0300-9084

Canani, RB, et al. (2011). Potential beneficial effects of butyrate in intestinal and extraintestinal diseases. *World Journal of Gastroenterology*, Vol. 17, No. 12, (Mar 2011), pp. (1519-1528), ISSN 1007-9327

Chassaing, B, et al. (2011). The commensal microbiota and enteropathogens in the pathogenesis of inflammatory bowel diseases. *Gastroenterology*, Vol. 140, No. 6, (May 2011), pp. (1720-1728), ISSN 1471-230X

Cherbut C, et al. (2003). The prebiotic characteristics of fructooligosaccharides are necessary for reduction of TNBS-induced colitis in rats. *The Journal of Nutrition*, Vol. 133, No. 1, (Jan 2003), pp. (21-27), ISSN 0022-3166

Coëffier, M, et al. (2010). Potential for amino acids supplementation during inflammatory bowel diseases. *Inflammatory Bowel Disease*, Vol. 16, No. 3, (March 2010), pp. (518-524), ISSN 1536-4844

Collado, MC, et al. (2009). The impact of probiotic on gut health. *Current Drug Metabolism*, Vol. 10, No. 1, (Jan 2009), pp. (68-78), ISSN 1389-2002

Corrao, G, et al. (1998). Risk of inflammatory bowel disease attributable to smoking, oral contraception and breastfeeding in Italy: a nationwide case-control study. Cooperative Investigators of the Italian Group for the Study of the Colon and the Rectum (GISC). *International Journal of Epidemiology*, Vol. 27, No. 3, (Jun 1998), pp. (397-404), ISSN 1464-3685

Cui, HH, et al. (2004). Effects of probiotic on intestinal mucosa of patients with ulcerative colitis. *World Journal of Gastroenterology*, Vol. 15, No. 10, (May 2004), pp. (1521-1525), ISSN 1007-9327

De Preter, V, et al. (2009). Pouchitis, similar to active ulcerative colitis, is associated with impaired butyrate oxidation by intestinal mucosa. *Inflammatory Bowel Disease*, Vol. 15, No. 3, (Mar 2009), pp. (335-340), ISSN 1536-4844

D'Haens, GR, et al. (1998). Early lesions of recurrent Crohn's disease caused by infusion of intestinal contents in excluded ileum. *Gastroenterology*, Vol. 114, No. 2, (Feb 1998), pp. (262-267), ISSN 1471-230X

Evaschuk, JB, et al. (2006). Probiotics and prebiotics in chronic inflammatory bowel diseases. *World Journal of Gastroenterology*, Vol. 12, No. 37, (Oct 2006), pp. (5941-5950), ISSN 1007-9327

Fava, F, & Danese, S. (2011). Intestinal microbiota in inflammatory bowel disease: Friend of foe? *World Journal of Gastroenterology*, Vol. 17, No. 5, (Feb 2011), pp. (557-566), ISSN 1007-9327

Ferguson, LR (2010). Nutrigenomics and inflammatory bowel diseases. *Expert review of Clinical Immunology*, Vol. 6, No. 4, (Jul 2010), pp. (573-583), 1744-666X

Fernandez-Banares, F, et al. (1999). Randomized clinical trial of Plantago ovata seeds (dietary fiber) as compared with mesalamine in maintaining remission in ulcerative colitis. *The American Journal of Gastroenterology*, Vol. 94, No. 2, (Feb 1999), pp. (427-433), ISSN 0002-9270

Furrie, E, et al. (2005). Synbiotic therapy (Bifidobacterium longum/Synergy 1) initiates resolution of inflammation in patients with active ulcerative colitis: a randomised controlled pilot trial. *Gut*, Vol. 54, No. 2, (Feb 2005), pp. (242-249), ISSN 0017-5749

Galli, C & Calder, PC. (2009). Effects of fat and fatty acid intake on inflammatory and immune responses: a critical review. *Annals of nutrition & metabolism*, Vol. 55, No. 1-3, (Sep 2009), pp. (123-139), ISSN 0250-6807

Geerling, BJ, et al. (2000). Diet as a risk factor for the development of ulcerative colitis. *The American Journal of Gastroenterology*, Vol. 95, No. 4, (Apr 2000), pp. (1008-1013), ISSN 0002-9270

Gionchetti, P, et al. (2000). Oral bacteriotherapy as maintenance treatment in patients with chronic pouchitis: a double-blind, placebo-controlled trial. *Gastroenterology*, Vol. 119, No. 2, (Aug 2000), pp. (305-309), ISSN 1471-230X

Gionchetti, P, et al. (2003). Prophylaxis of pouchitis onset with probiotic therapy: a double-blind placebo-controlled trial. *Gastroenterology*, Vol. 124, No. 5, (May 2003), pp. (1202-1209), ISSN 1471-230X

Guilloteau, P, et al. (2011). From the gut to the peripheral tissues: the multiple effects of butyrate. *Nutrition Research Reviews*, Vol. 23, No. 2, (Dec 2010), pp. (366-384), ISSN 0954-4224

Halfvarson, J, et al. (2003). Inflammatory bowel disease in a Swedish twin cohort: a long-term follow-up of concordance and clinical characteristics. *Gastroenterology*, Vol. 124, No. 7, (Jun 2003), pp. (1767-1773), ISSN 1471-230X

Hallert, C, et al. (1991). Ispaghula husk may relieve gastrointestinal symptoms in ulcerative colitis in remission. *Scandinavian Journal of Gastroenterology*, Vol. 26, No. 7, (Jul 1991), pp. (747-750), ISSN 0036-5521

Hallert, C, et al. (2003). Increasing fecal butyrate in ulcerative colitis patients by diet: controlled pilot study. *Inflammatory Bowel Disease*, Vol. 9, No. 2, (Mar 2003), pp. (116-121), ISSN 1536-4844

Hamer, HM, et al. (2008). Review article: the role of butyrate on colonic function. *Alimentary pharmacology & therapeutics*, Vol. 15, No. 2, (Jan 2008), pp. (104-119), ISSN 0269-2813

Hamer, HM, et al. (2010). Effect of butyrate enemas on inflammation and antioxidant status in the colonic mucosa of patients with ulcerative colitis in remission. *Clinical nutrition*, Vol. 29, No. 6, (Dec 2010), pp. (738-744), ISSN 0263-8290

Hanai, H, et al. (2004). Germinated barley foodstuff prolongs remission in patients with ulcerative colitis. *International Journal of Molecular Medicine*, Vol. 13, No. 5, (May 2004), pp. (643-647), ISSN 1791-244X

Hawthorne, AB, et al. (1992). Treatment of ulcerative colitis with fish oil supplementation: a prospective 12 month randomised controlled trial. *Gut*, Vol. 33, No. 7, (Jul 1992), pp. (922-928), ISSN 0017-5749

Holubar, SD, et al. (2010). Treatment and prevention of pouchitis after ileal pouch-anal anastomosis for chronic ulcerative colitis. *Cochrane database of systematic reviews*, Vol. 16, No. 6, (Jun 2010), pp. (CD001176), ISSN: 1469-493X

Hou JK, et al. (2011). Dietary intake and risk of developing inflammatory bowel disease: a systematic review of the literature. *The American Journal of Gastroenterology*, Vol. 106, No. 4, (Apr 2011), pp. (563-573), ISSN 0002-9270

Ioannidis, O, et al. (2011). Nutritional Modulation of the Inflammatory Bowel Response. *Digestion*, Vol. 84, No. 2, (Apr 1980), pp. (89-101), ISSN 0012-2823

Ishikawa, H, et al. (2003). Randomized controlled trial of the effect of bifidobacteria-fermented milk on ulcerative colitis. *Journal of the American College of Nutrition*, Vol. 22, No. 1, (Feb 2003), pp. (56-63), ISSN 0731-5724

Jeffery, NM, et al. (1997). Level of polyunsaturated fatty acids and the n-6 to n-3 polyunsaturated fatty acid ratio in the rat diet alter serum lipid levels and lymphocyte functions. *Prostaglandins Leukotriens Essentially Fatty Acids*, Vol. 57, No. 4-5, (Oct 1997), pp. (149–160), ISSN 0952-3278

Jijon, H, et al. (2004). DNA from probiotic bacteria modulates murine and human epithelial and immune function. *Gastroenterology*, Vol. 135, No. 7, (Jul 2005), pp. (1752-1756), ISSN 1471-230X

John, S, et al. (2010). Dietary n-3 polyunsaturated fatty acids and the aetiology of ulcerative colitis: a UK prospective cohort study. *European Journal of Gastroenterology and Hepatology*, Vol. 22, No. 5, (May 2010), pp. (243-249), ISSN 1473-56

Kanauchi, O, et al. (1999). Increased growth of Bifidobacterium and Eubacterium by germinated barley foodstuff, accompanied by enhanced butyrate production in healthy volunteers. *International Journal of Molecular Medicine*, Vol. 3, No. 2, (Feb 1999), pp. (175-179), ISSN 1791-244X

Kanauchi, O, et al. (2003). Germinated barley foodstuff, a prebiotic product, ameliorates inflammation of colitis through modulation of the enteric environment. *The Journal of Gastroenterology*, Vol. 38, No. 2, (Sep 2003), pp. (134-141), ISSN 0944-1174

Kanauchi, O, et al. (2003). Treatment of ulcerative colitis patients by long-term administration of germinated barley foodstuff: multi-center open trial. *International Journal of Molecular Medicine*, Vol. 12, No. 5, (Nov 2003), pp. (701-704), ISSN 1791-244X

Kato, K, et al. (2004). Randomized placebo-controlled trial assessing the effect of bifidobacteria-fermented milk on active ulcerative colitis. *Alimentary pharmacology & therapeutics*, Vol. 20, No. 10, (Nov 2004), pp. (1133-1141), ISSN 0269-2813

Klement, E, et al. (2004). Breastfeeding and risk of inflammatory bowel disease: a systematic review with meta-analysis. *The American Journal of Clinical Nutrition*, Vol. 80, No. 5, (Nov 2004), pp. (1342-1352), ISSN 0002-9165

Koletzko, S, et al. (1989). Role of infant feeding practices in development of Crohn's disease in childhood. *British Medical Journal*, Vol. 298, No. 6688, (Jun 1989), pp. (1617-1678), ISSN 0959-8138

Koletzko, S, et al. (1991). Infant feeding practices and ulcerative colitis in childhood. *British Medical Journal*, Vol. 302, No. 6792, (Jun 1991), pp. (1580-1581), ISSN 0959-8138

Kovarik, J, et al. (2011). Impaired anti-inflammatory efficacy of n-butyrate in patients with IBD. *European Journal of Clinical Investigation*, Vol. 41, No. 3, (Mar 2011), pp. (291-298), ISSN 1365-2362

Kruis, W, et al. (1997). Double-blind comparison of an oral Escherichia coli preparation and mesalazine in maintaining remission of ulcerative colitis. *Alimentary pharmacology & therapeutics*, Vol. 11, No. 5, (Oct 1997), pp. (853-858), ISSN 0269-2813

Kruis, W, et al. (2004). Maintaining remission of ulcerative colitis with the probiotic Escherichia coli Nissle 1917 is as effective as with standard mesalazine. *Gut*, Vol. 53, No. 11, (Nov 2004), pp. (1617-1623), ISSN 0017-5749

Kuisma, J, et al. (2003). Effect of Lactobacillus rhamnosus GG on ileal pouch inflammation and microbial flora. *Alimentary Pharmacology & Therapeutics*, Vol. 17, No. 4, (Feb 2003), pp. (509-515), ISSN 0269-2813

Li-Xuan, S, et al. (2010). Remission induction and maintenance effect of probiotics on ulcerative colitis: A meta-analysis. *World Journal of Gastroenterology*, Vol. 16, No. 15, (Apr 2010), pp. (1908-1915), ISSN 1007-9327

Lucendo, AJ & De Rezende, LC. (2009). Importance of nutrition in inflammatory bowel disease. *World Journal of Gastroenterology*, Vol. 15, No. 17, (May 2011), pp. (2081-2088), ISSN 1007-9327

Ma, D, et al. (2004). Live Lactobacillus reuteri is essential for the inhibitory effect on tumor necrosis factor alpha-induced interleukin-8 expression. *Infectiology and Immunology*, Vol. 72, No. 9, (Sep 2004), pp. (5308-5314), ISSN 0019-9567

Madsen, KL, et al. (1999). Lactobacillus species prevent colitis in interleukin 10 gene-deficient mice. *Gastroenterology*, Vol. 116, No. 5, (May 1999), pp. (1107-1114), ISSN 1471-230X

Mallon, DP & Suskind, DL (2010). Nutrition in pediatric inflammatory bowel disease. *Nutrition in Clinical Practice*, Vol. 25, No. 4, (Aug 2011), pp. (335-339), ISSN 0884-5336

Marteau, P. (2009). Bacterial flora in inflammatory bowel disease. *Journal of Digestive Diseases*, Vol. 27, No. 1, (Mar 2009), pp. (99-103), ISSN 1751-2980

Martini, GA, & Brandes, JW. (1976). Increased consumption of refined carbohydrates in patients with Crohn's disease. *Wiener klinische Wochenschrift*, Vol. 54, No. 8, (Apr 1976), pp. (367-371), ISSN 0043-5325

Miele, E, et al. (2009). Effect of a probiotic preparation (VSL#3) on induction and maintenance of remission in children with ulcerative colitis. *The American Journal of Gastroenterology*, Vol. 104, No. 2, (Feb 2009), pp. (437-443), ISSN 0002-9270

Mimura, T, et al. (2004). Once daily high dose probiotic therapy (VSL#3) for maintaining remission in recurrent or refractory pouchitis. *Gut*, Vol. 53, No. 1, (Jan 2004), pp. (108-114), ISSN 0017-5749

Otley, AR, et al. (2010). Nutritional therapy for the treatment of pediatric Crohn's disease. *Expert Review of Clinical Immunology*, Vol. 6, No. 4, (Jul 2010), pp. (667-676), 1744-666X

Persson, PG, et al. (1992). Diet and inflammatory bowel disease: a case-control study. *Epidemiology*, Vol. 3, No. 1, (Jan 1992), pp. (47-52), ISSN 1531-5487

Reif, S, et al. (2004). Pre-illness dietary factors in inflammatory bowel disease. *Gut*, Vol. 40, No. 6, (Jun 2004), pp. (754-760), ISSN 0017-5749

Rembacken, BJ, et al. (1999). Non-pathogenic Escherichia coli versus mesalazine for the treatment of ulcerative colitis: a randomised trial. *Lancet*, Vol. 354, No. 9179, (Aug 1999), pp. (771-774), ISSN 0140-6736

Roberfroid, M, et al. (2010). Prebiotic effects: metabolic and health benefits. *British Medical Journal*, Vol. 104, Suppl 2, (Aug 2010), pp. (S1-63), ISSN 0959-8138

Rose, DP, & Connolly, JM. (1999). Omega-3 fatty acids as cancer chemopreventive agents. *Pharmacology & Therapeutics*, Vol. 83, No. 3, (Sep 1999), pp. (217-244), ISSN 0163-7258

Russel, MG, et al. (1998). Modern life' in the epidemiology of inflammatory bowel disease: a case-control study with special emphasis on nutritional factors. *European Journal of Gastroenterology and Hepatology*, Vol. 10, No. 3, (Mar 1998), pp. (243-249), ISSN 1473-5687

Rutgeerts, P, et al. (1991). Effect of fecal stream diversion on the recurrence of Crohn's disease in a neoterminal ileum. *Lancet*, Vol. 338, No. 8770, (Sep 1997), pp. (771-774), ISSN 0140-6736

Sakamoto, N, et al. (2005). Epidemiology Group of the Research Committee on Inflammatory Bowel Disease in Japan. Dietary risk factors for inflammatory bowel disease: a multicenter case-control study in Japan. *Inflammatory Bowel Disease*, Vol. 11, No. 2, (Feb 2005), pp. (154-163), ISSN 1536-4844

Sartor, RB. (1997). The influence of normal microbial flora on the development of chronic mucosal inflammation. *Research in Immunology*, Vol. 148, No. 8-9, (Dec 1997), pp. (567-576), ISSN 0923-2494

Sartor, RB. (2004). Therapeutic manipulation of the enteric microflora in inflammatory bowel disease: antibiotics, probiotics and prebiotics. *Gastroenterology*, Vol. 126, No. 6, (May 2004), pp. (1620-1633), ISSN 1471-230X

Schirbel, A & Fiocchi, C. (2010). Inflammatory bowel disease: Established and evolving considerations on its etiopathogenesis and therapy. *Journal of Digestive Diseases*, Vol. 11, No. 5, (Oct 2010), pp. (266-726), ISSN 1751-2980

Schultz, M, et al. (2002). Lactobacillus plantarum 299V in the treatment and prevention of spontaneous colitis in interleukin-10-deficient mice. *Inflammatory Bowel Disease*, Vol. 8, No. 2, (Mar 2002), pp. (71-80), ISSN 1536-4844

Sellon, RK, (1998). Resident enteric bacteria are necessary for development of spontaneous colitis and immune system activation in interleukin-10-deficient mice. *Infectiology & Immunology*, Vol. 66, No. 11, (Nov 1998), pp. (5224-5231), ISSN 0019-9567

Sood, A, et al. (2009). The probiotic preparation, VSL#3 induces remission in patients with mild-to-moderately active ulcerative colitis. *Clinical Gastroenterology and Hepatology*, Vol. 7, No. 11, (Nov 2009), pp. (1202-1209), ISSN 1542-3565

Stange, EF, et al. (2008). The European consensus on ulcerative colitis: new horizons? Gut, Vol. 57, No. 8, (Aug 2008), pp. (1029-1931), ISSN 0017-5749

Stenson, WF, et al. (1992). Dietary supplementation with fish oil in ulcerative colitis. *Annals of Internal Medicine*, Vol. 116, No. 8, (Apr 1992), pp. (609-614), ISSN 1752-8526

Thomas, DW & Greer, FR. (2010). Probiotics and prebiotics in pediatrics. *Pediatrics*, Vol. 126, No.6, (Dec 2010), pp.(1217-1231), ISSN 1098-4275

Tjonneland, A, et al. (2009). Linoleic acid, a dietary n-6 polyunsaturated fatty acid, and the aetiology of ulcerative colitis: a nested case-control study within a European prospective cohort study. *Gut*, Vol. 58, No. 12, (Dec 2009), pp. (1606-1611), ISSN 0017-5749

Torres, MI & Ríos, A. (2008). Current view of the immunopathogenesis in inflammatory bowel disease and its implications for therapy. *World Journal of Gastroenterology*, Vol. 14, No. 13, (Apr 2008), pp. (1972-80), ISSN 1007-9327

Turner, D, et al. (2007). Omega 3 fatty acids (fish oil) for maintenance of remission in ulcerative colitis. *Cochrane database of systematic reviews*, Vol. 18, No. 3, (Jul 2007), pp. (CD006443), ISSN: 1469-493X

Turner, D, et al. (2011). Maintenance of remission in inflammatory bowel disease using omega-3 fatty acids (fish oil): a systematic review and meta-analyses. *Inflammatory Bowel Disease*, Vol. 17, No. 1, (Jan 2011), pp. (336-345), ISSN 1536-4844

Tursi, A, et al. (2004). Low-dose balsalazide plus a high-potency probiotic preparation is more effective than balsalazide alone or mesalazine in the treatment of acute mild-to-moderate ulcerative colitis. *Medical Science Monitor*, Vol. 10, No. 11, (Nov 2004), pp. (126-131), ISSN:1234-1010

Vernia, P, et al. (2003). Topical butyrate improves efficacy of 5-ASA in refractory distal ulcerative colitis: results of a multicentre trial. *European Journal of Clinical Investigation*, Vol. 33, No. 3, (Mar 2003), pp. (244-248), ISSN 1365-2362

Videla, S, et al. (2001). Dietary inulin improves distal colitis induced by dextran sodium sulfate in the rat. *The American Journal of Gastroenterology*, Vol. 96, No. 5, (May 2001), pp. (1486-1493), ISSN 0002-9270

Vieira de Barros, K, et al. (2011). Effects of a high fat or a balanced omega 3/omega 6 diet on cytokines levels and DNA damage in experimental colitis. *Nutrition*, Vol. 27, No. 2, (Feb 2011), pp. (221-226), ISSN 0899-9007

Zhang, L, et al. (2005). Alive and dead Lactobacillus rhamnosus GG decrease tumor necrosis factor-alpha-induced interleukin-8 production in Caco-2 cells. *The Journal of nutrition*, Vol. 135, No. 7, (Jul 2005), pp. (1752-1756), ISSN 0022-3166

Part 2

Special Population Groups

8

Ulcerative Colitis and Pregnancy

A. Alakkari and C. O'Morain
Adelaide and Meath Hospital,
Trinity College Dublin
Ireland

1. Introduction

Ulcerative Colitis (UC) is a chronic inflammatory condition that frequently affects men and women of childbearing age. Concerns are often raised by both patients and clinicians regarding the effects of the disease and its treatments on reproduction and lactation.

Many studies have examined fertility in UC patients in comparison with the general population. Most of these have not demonstrated a significant difference between the two groups. The observed decrease in fertility in some reports was largely attributable to patient choice, and the use of certain drugs such as sulfasalazine in men. Decreased fertility was also reported in women who have undergone surgery for their disease.

Pregnancy is considered high risk in patients with UC. Numerous studies have described the obstetric and neonatal outcomes of these patients, and reported similar pregnancy outcomes in comparison to the general population. However some population-based studies have found an increased incidence of low birth weight and preterm delivery in UC patients. This observed difference seems to be mainly related to disease activity and severity during pregnancy and the appropriate treatment required. On the other hand pregnancy does not appear to increase the risk of disease relapse or severity. The course of UC during pregnancy is partly determined by its activity at conception. Therefore UC patients should be advised to attempt to conceive during periods of disease remission.

Patients are often concerned about the safety of UC pharmacotherapy during pregnancy and lactation. Some patients choose to discontinue their maintenance therapy at least until the birth of their baby while others rely on their treating clinician to make the appropriate and safe decision regarding their treatment. Two issues have to be considered in this setting; first is the relative safety of the drug and secondly the benefit risk ratio of its use in pregnancy and lactation. A large amount of safety data is available on drugs that have been in use for decades, however modern medicine has witnessed the introduction of new therapeutic agents that have revolutionized the treatment of inflammatory diseases but there is limited data available regarding their safety during pregnancy and breast feeding.

The topic of UC and pregnancy is quite complex involving a range of issues including the effects of both the disease and its treatment options on fertility, pregnancy and lactation, in addition to the effects of pregnancy and lactation on the course of the disease. The aim of this chapter is to review the available data and discuss this topic in more detail.

2. UC and fertility

There are a number of considerations when discussing the relationship between UC and fertility including the effects of the disease and the medical and surgical management options on both male and female reproduction and the risk of infertility. Infertility is defined as failure to conceive after one year of regular unprotected intercourse.

A number of studies have suggested that male fertility in UC is comparable to the general population. A survey of 62 men with UC and 140 controls found the number of pregnancies in the UC group was not statistically different to that in the control group. Fecundability (the probability of pregnancy per menstrual cycle with unprotected intercourse) was similar in the two groups [1]. A case control study of 1400 patients by Moody et al demonstrated no significant difference in the mean number of children born to male patients with UC compared to the general population [2].

Fertility rates decline in male patients following ileal pouch anal anastomosis (IPAA) for UC. In a retrospective review of 111 patients by Heuting et al [3] the incidence of sexual dysfunction after IPAA was reported at 20%. A smaller prospective study of 18 patients by Berndtsson et al [4] showed loss of ejaculation in <5% of male patients following IPAA. However in both studies the patients reported overall satisfaction with their quality of life including overall sexual function following surgery. Gorgun et al assessed sexual function in 122 male patients who underwent IPAA between 1995 -2000 using the validated International Index of Erectile Function (IIEF) scoring instrument. This index scale examines sexual function in five categories: erectile function, orgasmic function, sexual desire, intercourse satisfaction and overall satisfaction. There was a statistically significant improvement in the scores of 4 categories following surgery with an increase in the mean erectile function score by 2.12 points (p=0.02) after IPAA [5].

Initial studies demonstrated infertility rates of up to 49% among women with UC, which is higher than documented for the general population (7%-12%)[6]. More recent studies have shown that female UC patients who have not had surgery have fertility rates comparable to the general population, and this largely reflects improvement in the medical management of UC over the years, leading to better control of disease activity, general health and reproductive function. In a study comparing 290 women with UC to 661 non IBD controls, Olsen et al found equal fecundability ratios (FR=1.01) in the two groups, but FR dropped to 0.02 (p<0.001) after IPAA, figure 1 demonstrates the results of the study [7]. Johnson et al confirmed these findings in a study showing 13.3% infertility rates in UC patients who are medically managed compared to 38.6% infertility rates in UC patients following IPAA, p<0.001 [8].

2.1 Drugs used for UC and fertility

Medical management of UC involves the use of a range of pharmacological agents with variable effects on fertility in males and females. Sulphasalazines and 5-aminosalicylates (5ASA) are often used for maintenance of disease remission in UC. Both rat and human studies have demonstrated reduced male fertility during the use of sulphasalazine due to its adverse effects on sperm count, morphology and motility. These effects are secondary to the non-therapeutic sulphapyridine moiety and are completely reversible on cessation of the drug [9,10], or replacing it with a different 5ASA [11]. There are no reports of reduced female fertility with the use of sulphasalazine.

Corticosteroids are used to induce remission during exacerbations of UC. They have been shown in rat studies to depress serum testosterone levels, but have no effect on gonadotropin levels [12]. Serum testosterone levels returned to normal on withdrawal of steroid treatment. Lerman et al demonstrated similar effects on fertility in male rats, although no change was seen in sperm number and motility [13]. There is limited data on the effects of exogenous steroids on male fertility in humans. A study by Roberts et al, suggested that an increase in endogenous cortisol levels observed following strenuous exercise was associated with a subsequent decrease in sperm concentration [14]. Therefore, steroids should only be used short term to control disease activity. The use of steroids for different diseases in females has not been associated with impaired fertility.

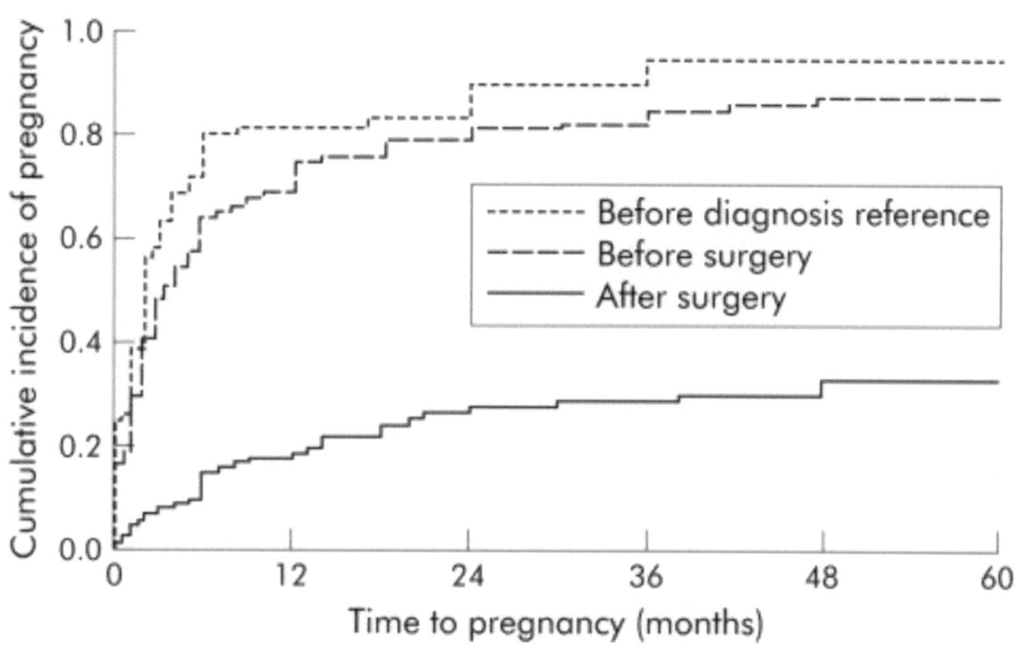

Fig. 1. Fecundability ratio in patients with ulcerative colitis before and after diagnosis, and after ileal pouch anal anastomosis compared with healthy controls. Reprinted from Olsen and colleagues [7]

Immunosuppressants are frequently used in the management of UC as steroid-sparing drugs to maintain disease remission. Their effects on male fertility in humans are controversial. Although the use of Mercaptopurine (MP) in male mice has been associated with reduce fertility [15], it has not been shown to affect sperm count or quality [16]. Francella et al, in a retrospective review of 485 IBD male and female patients found that the use of MP did not result in a statistically significant difference in conception failure compared to IBD patients not receiving MP [17]. Review of the long-term use of immunosuppressants such as Azathioprine in renal transplant patients has also shown no obvious effects on fertility in both males and females [18].

The use of anti-TNFα agents in the management of UC has been increasing over the last decade with accumulating evidence to support its beneficial effects. There are no human data on the effects of biologic therapy on fertility but data on its safety during pregnancy is increasing (this will be discussed in more detail later). Animal studies have demonstrated no adverse effects on both male and female fertility [19].

3. UC and pregnancy

3.1 The effects of UC on pregnancy

Pregnancy is considered high risk in patients with UC, and this is primarily related to disease activity at conception and during pregnancy. The overall outcome of pregnancy in UC is comparable to the general population however active disease during pregnancy especially when severe results in adverse pregnancy outcomes. This has been confirmed by a number of studies. A Danish population based study demonstrated no increased risk of low birth weight and intrauterine growth retardation in patients with UC, however the risk of preterm delivery was increased when the first hospitalization for UC took place during pregnancy (odds ratio = 3.4, 95% confidence interval = 1.8-6.4) [20]. A retrospective review of 98 pregnancies in IBD patients by Federkow et al, found a statistically significant higher rate of preterm delivery ($p < 0.01$) than the rate of the control group. The risk was further increased when a disease exacerbation occurred during pregnancy [21]. Bush et al, in a case control study of 116 pregnancies in IBD patients demonstrated an increased risk of low birth weight in the UC group compared to the Crohn's disease (CD) group (19% vs. 0%, $p = 0.002$), with flares during pregnancy associated with an increased risk for preterm delivery (27% vs. 8%, $p = 0.02$) and LBW (32% vs. 3%, $p = 0.003$) [22]. A population based cohort study of 239773 pregnant women including 756 women with IBD, by Kornfeld et al, supported the increased risk of adverse pregnancy outcomes such as preterm delivery, low birth weight, small for gestational age, and cesarean section in pregnant women with IBD [23]. Therefore control of disease activity during pregnancy is imperative for the well being of the mother and the baby.

3.2 The effects of pregnancy on UC

Pregnancy was initially thought to lead to improved control of disease activity during the gestational period as a result of the relative suppression of the mother's immune system to allow fetal development. However, evidence suggests that gestational disease activity is influenced by factors other than the physiological state of pregnancy. Disease activity during pregnancy is determined by activity at conception. Patients who conceive during disease remission have relapse rates comparable to non-pregnant UC patients over a nine-month period, with 70-80% of these patients remaining in remission throughout the gestational period [24]. If an exacerbation occurs it is likely to be mild and responsive to medical treatment. In patients with active disease at conception, about 45% will deteriorate, 25% will improve and 25% will remain unchanged, therefore about 3 out of 4 will have active disease during their pregnancy, resulting in adverse perinatal outcomes [24].

The risk of postpartum disease relapse is partly determined by disease activity at the time of delivery. In a study of 324 patients, Modagam et al demonstrated that only 13% of patients with quiescent to mild disease at term experienced a flare in the puerperal period in contrast to 53% of patients with active disease at delivery [25]. However, there is evidence suggesting that pregnancy itself leads to improved control of IBD activity in the years following it. Castiglione et al reported reduced rates of disease relapse in the first three years after pregnancy compared to the pre-pregnancy period in UC patients ($p<0.005$) [26].

Pregnancy is safe in patients with IPAA but impaired pouch function can be experienced during pregnancy with increased daytime and nocturnal stool frequency and incontinence. However, pouch function tends to return to pre-pregnancy function following delivery [27].

3.3 Mode of delivery in UC

The observed rates of caesarean section in UC is higher than the general population [27]. The reason for this is unknown. The decision to proceed to cesarean section should be made purely on obstetric grounds except in cases where the patient has undergone IPAA. Such patients can have normal vaginal deliveries without damaging the pouch [28], however there is concern for damage to the anal sphincter. The risk of anal sphincter damage is compounded by aging, therefore the effects may not become apparent for several years. Although the current reports of IPAA patients who have had vaginal deliveries demonstrate no irreversible pouch complications in the majority of patients, there is no long-term follow-up data available (i.e. 20-30 years). Therefore, the decision on mode of delivery in IPAA patients should be made following detailed discussion of the potential effects on pouch and anal function by the patient, obstetrician and colorectal surgeon.

3.4 Medications for the treatment in UC and pregnancy

Patients are often concerned about the potential teratogenecity of the drugs used in UC and may even opt to discontinue their maintenance therapy during pregnancy. Experience and data support the safe use of many maintenance drugs during pregnancy. In fact, disease relapses and continued disease activity during pregnancy as a result of either cessation of maintenance therapy or/and avoiding induction therapy are more harmful to both the mother and the unborn baby [29]. Patients should be counseled prior to pregnancy regarding the potential toxicity of some of their medications, however they should be advised to maintain safe medical treatment for adequate control of disease activity during pregnancy. The risk of maternal drug exposure to fetal development is classified by the Food and Drug Administration (FDA) into categories, see table 1. The FDA pregnancy categories of drugs used in UC are summarized in table 2.

5 Aminosalicylates & sulphasalazine

5 ASA preparations are frequently used as first line maintenance therapy for UC. They have been in use for decades with numerous studies supporting their safe use in pregnant patients. The FDA currently classifies them as pregnancy category B. Although 5 ASAs are poorly absorbed from the gastrointestinal tract, they do cross the placenta once they reach systemic circulation [30]. No consistent teratogenic effect has been demonstrated in animal and human studies. In a prospective cohort study of 60 pregnant IBD patients, Norgard et al found no substantial increased risk of malformations in patients who received 5ASAs during the first trimester of pregnancy, odds ratio 1.9 (95% confidence interval 0.7-5.4) [31], but observed an increased risk of stillbirths and preterm deliveries which could be due to the disease rather than the drugs as the controls used were women without IBD. A meta-analysis of 7 studies, that included 2200 pregnant women with IBD; 642 received 5-ASA

drugs (mesalazine, sulfasalazine or olsalazine) and 1158 received no medication, suggested only a 1.16-fold increase in congenital malformations, a 2.38-fold increase in stillbirth, a 1.14-fold increase in spontaneous abortion, a 1.35-fold increase in preterm delivery, and a 0.93-fold increase in low birth weight [32].

FDA Pharmaceutical Pregnancy Categories	
Pregnancy Category A	Adequate and well-controlled human studies have failed to demonstrate a risk to the fetus in the first trimester of pregnancy (and there is no evidence of risk in later trimesters).
Pregnancy Category B	Animal reproduction studies have failed to demonstrate a risk to the fetus and there are no adequate and well-controlled studies in pregnant women OR Animal studies have shown an adverse effect, but adequate and well-controlled studies in pregnant women have failed to demonstrate a risk to the fetus in any trimester.
Pregnancy Category C	Animal reproduction studies have shown an adverse effect on the fetus and there are no adequate and well-controlled studies in humans, but potential benefits may warrant use of the drug in pregnant women despite potential risks.
Pregnancy Category D	There is positive evidence of human fetal risk based on adverse reaction data from investigational or marketing experience or studies in humans, but potential benefits may warrant use of the drug in pregnant women despite potential risks.
Pregnancy Category X	Studies in animals or humans have demonstrated fetal abnormalities and/or there is positive evidence of human fetal risk based on adverse reaction data from investigational or marketing experience, and the risks involved in use of the drug in pregnant women clearly outweigh potential benefits.

Table 1. FDA drug category during pregnancy

FDA B	FDA C	FDA D	FDA X
5 ASAs Amoxicillin/ Clav Metronidazole Infliximab Adalimumab	Corticosteroids Ciprofloxacin Cyclosporin Loperamide	Azathioprine Mercaptopurine Lomotil	Methotrexate

Table 2. FDA pregnancy category of drugs used for UC

Sulfasalazine was initially thought to be teratogenic, however more recent studies failed to identify significant association between the drug and congenital anomalies [33, 34]. Sulfasalazine interacts with the cell membrane transporter for natural folates and interferes with folate absorption, which in turn may lead to folate deficiency with increased risk of neural tube defects and cardiovascular defects [35, 36]. Therefore folate supplementation with up to 2mg of folic acid daily should be strongly recommended to female patients on sulfalazine even prior to pregnancy [37]. Alternatively, patients could be switched to mesalamine, but they should still be advised to take 400micrograms of folic acid daily when planning to conceive.

Corticosteroids

Corticosteroids are indicated for induction of disease remission during exacerbations of UC. The FDA classifies them as pregnancy category C. Their use in pregnancy has been associated with increased risk of cleft palate in a number of case control studies [38, 39]. In a prospective control study of 311 pregnant IBD patients, Gur et al found no significant difference in the rate of major anomalies between the group treated with corticosteroids (GCS) during pregnancy compared to the control group [12/262 = 4.6% (GCS), 19/728 = 2.6% (control), [P = 0.116]. There was no case of oral cleft and no pattern of anomalies among the GCS exposed group [40].

Corticosteroids can cross the placenta but the rate varies with the type of steroid depending on the extent of placental metabolism and placental and albumin binding affinity [41]. Fetal exposure to prednisolone is lower than for other steroids such as dexamethasone, and should therefore be used in preference to them during pregnancy [42, 43].

Immunosuppressants

Escalation of maintenance medical treatment to immunosuppressants is required in patients with moderate to severe refractory UC. This category includes azathioprine (AZA), mercaptopurines (MP), and methotrexate (MTX). The first two drugs are classified by the FDA as category D drugs, but MTX is classified as category X, and patients should be advised not to conceive on the drug or even within 3 months of stopping it, as it is associated with a high risk of developing craniofacial deformities, limb defects and severe central nervous system abnormalities [44].

AZA/MP are relatively less toxic during pregnancy in humans although animal studies have demonstrated an increased risk of teratogenecity with their use [15]. The oral bioavailability of the two drugs is low (47% for AZA and 16% for MP)(44), and their placental transfer is limited [45]. AZA/MP are absorbed in their inactive form and the fetal liver lacks the enzyme necessary to convert them to the active and potentially toxic metabolites [46]. Case reports of the teratogenic effects of AZA use during pregnancy such as chromosomal abnormalities and myelotoxicity in the infant originate from transplant and oncology patients using higher doses of the drug than would be used in UC [47]. AZA is used at a dose of 1-1.5mg/kg of body weight in patients with UC, and studies on its effects during pregnancy at this dose have found no increased risk of teratogenicity [48- 50]. In a large retrospective review of 325 pregnancies, Francella et al showed that the use of AZA/ MP prior to, at conception and during pregnancy does not increase the risk of spontaneous abortions, stillbirths, prematurity or the rate of neonatal or childhood infections [17]. Shim et al reported the safe use of AZA /MP in pregnant IBD patients in Australia. In 19 births exposed to AZA /MP there was 1 neonatal adverse outcome in the exposed group as compared to 4 in controls (5.3% vs. 5.4%, p=0.97). One congenital anomaly was seen in each group (p=0.27). No low birth weight at term was seen in either group. Placental blood flow in 4 women exposed to AZA /MP was normal [51]. In a large cohort from the CESAME study, Coelho et al found no significant difference in overall pregnancy outcomes between pregnancies exposed to thiopurines (n=86) and those not exposed to any treatment (n=45) [52].

Cyclosporin (CYA) is indicated in patients with fulminant colitis or severe exacerbations of UC unresponsive to induction therapy with steroids. It is classified as FDA category C. It is only 34% absorbed from the gastrointestinal tract, but can cross the placenta [53]. Animal studies found some fetal toxicity associated with exposure to the drug at maternotoxic doses including embryo lethality, and reduced fetal growth [54]. Reports of its use in humans during pregnancy come from transplant patients. A meta-analysis of 15 studies that included 410 patients failed to identify any significant teratogenicity associated with the use of CYA. The rates of prematurity and low birth weight were higher in infants exposed to CYA, but did not reach statistical significance [55]. In cases of fulminant colitis the use of CYA may preclude the need for colectomy. Colectomy resulted in fetal loss in 2 of 4 pregnant patients who underwent surgery for fulminant colitis in a case series by Anderson et al [56].

Biologic agents

Anti TNFα therapy was initially used in refractory and fistulating CD, but there is increasing evidence to support its use in UC. Naturally there were numerous concerns for their potential toxicity in pregnancy, however recent studies have demonstrated their safety during pregnancy. A case series of 4 pregnant IBD patients who continued their infliximab (IFX) treatment during pregnancy by Zolinkova et al, reported therapeutic IFX levels in the cord blood of 3 babies at levels 2-3 fold higher than in the peripheral blood of the their mothers, and during the 3- to 6-month follow-up, the children developed normally without signs of infections or allergic reactions, and had normal antibody titres after routine childhood vaccinations [57]. A larger observational study by Schnitzler et al, assessed 212 IBD patients on anti TNFα treatment and found that 32 of the 42 pregnancies ended in live births with a median gestational age of 38 weeks (interquartile range [IQR] 37-39). There were seven premature deliveries, six children had low birth weight, and there was one stillbirth. One boy weighed 1640 g delivered at week 33, died at age 13 days secondary to necrotizing enterocolitis. A total of eight abortions (one patient wish) occurred in seven women. Trisomy 18 was diagnosed in one foetus of a mother with CD at age 37 years under adalimumab (ADA) treatment (40 mg weekly) and pregnancy was terminated. Pregnancy outcomes after direct exposure to anti-TNFα treatment were not different from those in pregnancies before anti-TNFα treatment or with indirect exposure to anti-TNFα treatment but outcomes were worse than in pregnancies before IBD diagnosis [58]. Anti TNFα drugs are classified as pregnancy category B by the FDA.

Although data supports the safe use of biologic therapy in UC patients during pregnancy, we must be aware of the potential complications of immunosuppression in babies born to mothers receiving anti TNFα treatment during the third trimester of pregnancy. Cheent et al reported a case of an infant born to a mother who received IFX throughout her pregnancy, dying of disseminated TB infection at age 4.5 months after receiving BCG vaccination at the age of 3 months. Live attenuated vaccines including BCG are contraindicated in individuals who are receiving immunosuppressive drugs, and physicians should exercise caution before such vaccines are used in infants born to mothers taking anti-TNF therapies or other potentially immunosuppressive IgG1 antibodies [59]. Consideration should be given to the cessation of biologic treatment in the third trimester of pregnancy to reduce foetal exposure to the drug immediately prior to delivery.

Antibiotics

Antibiotics such as metronidazole and ciprofloxacin have limited use in UC. Their short-term use for the treatment of pouchitis post IPAA is considered low risk in pregnancy. Metronidazole is classified as FDA pregnancy category B. Its use in pregnancy has not been associated with increased risk of congenital abnormalities. A retrospective review by Sorensen et al demonstrated no increased preterm delivery following metronidazole treatment during pregnancy in a cohort of 124 patients [60]. Diav-Citrin et al prospective studied 228 women exposed to metronidazole during pregnancy and found no significant difference between the cases and controls in terms of congenital abnormalities and preterm delivery, however the mean birth weight was lower in the treatment group [61]. Amoxicillin/ clavulanic acid is an FDA category B drug and is considered safe during pregnancy.

Ciprofloxacin and other quinolones are classified as FDA pregnancy category C drugs. In a prospective review of 200 patients treated with quinolones during pregnancy, Loebstein et al failed to show an increased risk of arthropathy demonstrated in animal studies [62]. There was no significant increased rate of spontaneous abortions, prematurity or birth weight in the treatment group. Sulphonamides and tetracyclines are contraindicated in pregnancy.

Anti-diarrheals

Anti-diarrheal agents are used for symptomatic relief during pregnancy. Loperamide is classified as FDA category B drug. In a prospective case control study of 105 women, Einarson et al found no increased risk of miscarriage, preterm delivery or congenital anomalies with the use of loperamide intermittently during pregnancy [63]. However, a Lower mean birth weight was documented in infants whose mothers received loperamide continuously during pregnancy. Another study of 638 pregnancies exposed to loperamide from early pregnancy showed an increased rate of congenital defects (OR 1.41; 97% CI 1.03 - 1.93); only hypospadias showed a significant increase (RR=3.2, 95% CI 1.3 - 6.6) [64]. Lomotil (diphenoxylate hydrochloride/atropine) is classified as FDA category C drug. It should be used with caution in pregnant patients, as it is not known whether it can cross the placenta.

4. UC and breastfeeding

Breastfeeding has well-recognized benefits to infants, including reducing the risk of developing IBD in later life [65]. It has not been shown to influence the pattern of UC disease activity in the post partum period [66]. However, patients are often concerned about the potential toxicity of pharmacological UC therapy to the breastfed infant. Patients should be offered individual advice regarding whether or not to breastfeed depending on the benefit/ risk ratio of the prescribed medication on the infant, and the risk of cessation of medical therapy to the mother.

Sulphasalazine and other 5ASAs are relatively safe during breastfeeding as less than 10% of the maternal dose is excreted in breast milk [67], however there are two case reports in the literature describing diarrhea in a breastfed infant whose mother was being treated with sulphasalazine [68, 69]. There are no other studies demonstrating adverse effects of 5ASAs on breastfed infants, therefore UC patients should be encouraged to breastfeed while on aminosalicylates.

Only 5 - 25 % of maternal plasma steroid concentrations are present in breast milk [70], therefore infant exposure to the drug is very low. There are no reports of harmful effects on infants breastfed by mothers taking corticosteroids, however patients should be advised to delay breastfeeding by 4 hours following administration of steroids to decrease infant exposure to the drug since its half life is 3 hours [71].

Immunosuppressants are secreted in breast milk and can potentially suppress the infant's immune system. Clinical experience suggests that AZA and MP are safe to use while breastfeeding. In a retrospective review of nursing mothers taking AZA, Angelberger et al demonstrated that the infants had age appropriate mental status and physical development compared to the control group with no difference in the rate of hospitalization [72]. CYA and MTX should be avoided by nursing mothers due to the risk of infant immunosuppression, potential harmful effects on growth, and association with carcinogenesis [73]. There is limited data describing the use of biologic drugs during lactation. In a small case series of 3 mothers treated with IFX during the post partum period, Kane et al found no detectable levels of IFX in the breast milk or the sera of the breastfed infants [74]. This suggests that mothers on IFX should not be discouraged from breastfeeding. It is not known whether ADA is secreted in breast milk and should therefore be avoided in nursing mothers.

Amoxicillin/ clavulanic acid is safe to use in nursing mothers [75], however there is limited data regarding metronidazole and ciprofloxacin, and they should be avoided during breastfeeding. Loperamide and diphenoxylate hydrochloride are excreted in breast milk and should be avoided in nursing mothers [70]. See table 3 for the summary of drug safety during breastfeeding.

Low risk	**Limited data**	**Not recommended**	**Contraindicated**
Steroids Mesalamine Sulphasalazine Amoxicillin/ clavulanic acid	Adalimumab Infliximab	Metronidazole Ciprofloxacin Azathioprine Mercaptopurine	Methotrexate Cyclosporin

Table 3. Safety of drugs during breastfeeding

5. Summary

Patients with UC should be reassured that the diagnosis of UC does not necessarily imply impaired fertility and/or increased risk of congenital and developmental abnormalities in the baby. Impaired fertility is related to disease activity, pharmacological agents used for medical management, and/or surgery for UC (IPAA). Active UC at conception is associated with increased risk of gestational disease activity and exacerbations, which in turn is associated with increased risk of adverse pregnancy outcomes. Although certain drugs used for the treatment of UC such as MTX are potentially teratogenic and are contraindicated prior to and during pregnancy, the majority of them are relatively safe, including immunosuppressants and biologic agents. Clinical experience has demonstrated that disease activity during pregnancy is more harmful to both the mother and the baby than the majority of drugs used to treat exacerbations, and /or maintain remission of UC during pregnancy.

UC patients should be advised to attempt to conceive during periods of disease remission. The potential toxicity of medical treatment in pregnancy should be discussed, and the benefit / risk ratio estimated on an individual basis.

UC patients should not be discouraged from breastfeeding their infants, however the potential toxicity of the mother's medications should be taken into consideration and the risk to the baby weighed against the risk of disease relapse in the mother if medical treatment was discontinued.

6. Expert opinion

The second European evidence-based consensus on the diagnosis and management of inflammatory bowel disease (IBD) published the following statements in relation to IBD and pregnancy [76]:

IBD and fertility:

- IBD does not seem to affect fertility when the disease is inactive, however disease activity leads to reduced fertility.
- Female patients who undergo surgery are at risk of impaired tubal function.
- In male patients rectal excision may cause impotence of ejaculatory problems, however there is no comparison with the general population.
- Sulphasalazine therapy causes reversible infertility in male patients because of changes in semen quality.

IBD and pregnancy:

- It is advisable to strive for clinical remission before conception.
- If conception occurs at a time of quiescent disease the risk of relapse is the same as on non-pregnant women.
- If conception occurs at a time of disease activity, two thirds have persistent activity, and of these two thirds deteriorate.
- Flares are best treated aggressively to prevent complications.
- Insufficient data exists about maternal morbidity and fetal mortality at surgery.
- Both clinical activity and surgical intervention decline with pregnancy and parity.

Mode of delivery:

- The mode of delivery should primarily be governed by obstetric necessity and indication, but also in conjunction with the gastroenterologist and/or colorectal surgeon.
- An ileo-anal pouch is regarded as an indication for caesarean section.
- Colostomy or ileostomy patients can deliver vaginally.

Medical treatment during pregnancy:

- Medical treatment for IBD should generally continue during pregnancy, because the benefits outweigh the risk of medication.

7. References

[1] Narendranathan M, Sandler RS, Suchindran CM, et al. Male infertility in inflammatory bowel disease. *J Clin Gastroenterol* 1989;11:403–6.

[2] Moody GA, Probert C, Jayanthi V, Mayberry JF. The effects of chronic ill health and treatment with sulphasalazine on fertility amongst men and women with inflammatory bowel disease in Leicestershire. *Int J Colorectal Dis* 1997; 12: 220–4.
[3] Hueting WE, Gooszen HG, Van Laarhoven CJ. Sexual function and continence after ileo pouch anal anastomosis: a comparison between a meta-analysis and a questionnaire survey. *Int J Colorectal Dis* 2004; 19: 215–8.
[4] Berndtsson I, Oresland T, Hulten L. Sexuality in patients with ulcerative colitis before and after restorative proctocolectomy: a prospective study. *Scand J Gastroenterol* 2004; 39: 374–9.
[5] Gorgun E, Remzi FH, Montague DK, Connor JT, O'Brien K, Loparo B, Fazio VW. Male sexual function improves after ileal pouch anal anastomosis. *Colorectal Dis.* 2005 Nov;7(6):545-50.
[6] De Dombal FT, Watts JM, Watkinson G, Goligher JC. Ulcerative colitis and pregnancy. *Lancet* 1965; 25: 599–602.
[7] Olsen KO, Juul S, Berndtsson I, et al. Ulcerative colitis: female fecundity before diagnosis, during disease, and after surgery compared with a population sample. *Gastroenterology* 2002;122:15–19.
[8] Johnson P, Richard C, Ravid A, et al. Female infertility after ileal pouch-anal anastomosis for ulcerative colitis. *Dis Colon Rectum* 2004;47:1119–26.
[9] Levi AJ, Fisher AM, Hughes L, Henry WF. Male infertility due to sulphasalazine. *Lancet* 1979; 314:276–8.
[10] O'Morain C, Smethurst P, Dore CJ, Levi AJ. Reversible male infertility due to sulphasalazine: studies in man and rat. *Gut* 1984; 25:1078–84.
[11] Zelissen PM, Van Hattum J, Poen H, Scholten P, Gerritse R, Te Velde ER. Influence of salazosulphapyridine and 5-aminosalicylic acid on seminal qualities and male sex hormones. *Scand J Gastroenterol* 1988; 23: 1100–4
[12] Balasubramanian K, Aruldhas MM, Govindarajulu P. Effect of corticosterone on rat epididymal lipids. *J Androl* 1987; 8: 69–73.
[13] Lerman SA, Miller GK, Bohlman K, et al. Effects of corticosterone on reproduction in male Sprague-Dawley rats. *Reprod Toxicol* 1997; 11: 799- 805.
[14] Roberts AC, McClure RD, Weiner RI, Brooks GA. Overtraining affects male reproductive status. *Fertil Steril* 1993; 60: 686–92.
[15] Polifka JE, Friedman JM. Teratogen update: azathioprine and 6- mercaptopurine. *Teratology* 2002;65:240-61.
[16] Dejaco C, Mittermaier C, Reinisch W, et al. Azathioprine treatment and male fertility in inflammatory bowel disease. *Gastroenterology* 2001; 121: 1048–53.
[17] Francella A, Dyan A, Bodian C, Rubin P, Chapman M, Present DH. The safety of 6-mercaptopurine for childbearing patients with inflammatory bowel disease: a retrospective cohort study. *Gastroenterology* 2003; 124: 9–17.
[18] Xu L, Han S, Liu Y, Wang H, et al. The influence of immunosuppressants on the fertility of males who undergo renal transplantation and on the immune function of their offspring. Transpl Immunol. 2009 Dec;22(1-2):28-31.
[19] Treacy G. Using an analogous monoclonal antibody to evaluate the reproductive and chronic toxicity potential for a humanized anti-TNF-a monoclonal antibody. *Hum Exp Toxicol* 2000;19: 226–8.

[20] Norgard B, Fonager K, Sorensen H T. et al Birth outcomes of women with ulcerative colitis: a nationwide Danish cohort study. *Am J Gastroenterol* 2000. 953165–3170.

[21] Fedorkow D M, Persaud D, Nimrod C A. Inflammatory bowel disease: a controlled study of late pregnancy outcome. *Am J Obstet Gynecol* 1989. 160998–1001.

[22] Bush M C, Patel S, Lapinski R H. et al Perinatal outcomes in inflammatory bowel disease. *J Matern Fetal Neonatal Med* 2004. 15237–241.

[23] Kornfeld D, Cnattingius S, Ekbom A. Pregnancy outcomes in women with inflammatory bowel disease—a population-based cohort study. *Am J Obstet Gynecol* 1997. 177942–946.

[24] Miller JP. Inflammatory bowel disease in pregnancy: a review. *J R Soc Med* 1986;79:221-5.

[25] Mogadam M, Korelitz BI, Ahmed SW, Dobbins WO, 3rd, Baiocco PJ. The course of inflammatory bowel disease during pregnancy and post partum. *Am J Gastroenterol* 1981a; 75: 265–9.

[26] Castiglione F, et al. Effect of pregnancy on the clinical course of a cohort of women with inflammatory bowel disease. Ital J Gastroenterol. 1996 May;28(4):199-204.

[27] Ravid A, Richard CS, Spencer LM, et al. Pregnancy, delivery and pouch function after ileal pouch-anal anastomosis for ulcerative colitis. *Dis Colon Rectum* 2002; 45: 1283–8.

[28] Juhasz ES, Fozard B, Dozois RR, Ilstrup DM, Nelson H. Ileal pouch-anal anastomosis function following childbirth: an extended evaluation. *Dis Colon Rectum* 1995; 38: 159–65.

[29] Moffatt DC, Bernstein CN. Drug therapy for inflammatory bowel disease in pregnancy and the puerperium. Best Pract Res Clin Gastroenterol. 2007;21(5):835-47.

[30] Christensen LA, Rasmussen SN, Hansen SH. Disposition of 5-aminosalicylic Acid and N-acetyl-5-aminosalicylic acid in fetal and maternal body-fluids during treatment with different 5-aminosalicylic acid preparations. Acta Obstet Gynecol Scand, 1994;73:399-40.

[31] Norgard B, Fonager K, Pedersen L, et al. Birth outcome in women exposed to 5-aminosalicylic acid during pregnancy: a Danish cohort. study Gut 2003;52:243-7.

[32] Rahimi R, Nikfar S, Rezaie A, et al. Pregnancy outcome in women with inflammatory bowel disease following exposure to 5-aminosalicylic acid drugs: a meta-analysis. Reprod Toxicol2008;25:271-5.

[33] Hoo JJ, Hadro TA, Von Behren P. Possible teratogenicity of sulfasalazine. N Engl J Med 1988;318:1128.

[34] Norgard B, Czeizel AE, Rockenbauer M, et al. Population-based case control study of the safety of sulfasalazine use during pregnancy. Aliment Pharmacol Ther, 2001;15:483-6.

[35] Jansen G, Van der Heijden J, Oerlemans R, et al. Sulfasalazine is a potent inhibitor of the reduced folate carrier: implications for combination therapies with methotrexate in rheumatoid arthritis. Arthritis Rheum 2004; 50: 2130–9.

[36] Czeizel AE, Toth M, Rockenbauer M. Population-based case control study of folic acid supplementation during pregnancy.Teratology 1996; 53: 645–51.

[37] Mahadevan U, Kane S. American Gastroenterological Association Institute Technical Review on the use of gastrointestinal medications in pregnancy. *Gastroenterology* 2006; 131: 283–311.

[38] Rodriguez-Pinilla E, Martinez-Frias ML. Corticosteroids during pregnancy and oral clefts: a case-control study. Teratology 1998;58: 2–5.

[39] Carmichael SL, Shaw GM. Maternal corticosteroid use and risk of selected congenital anomalies. Am J Med Genet 1999; 86:242–4.

[40] Gur C, Diav-Citrin O, Shechtman S, Arnon J, Ornoy A. Pregnancy outcome after first trimester exposure to corticosteroids: a prospective controlled study. *Reprod Toxicol* 2004; 18: 93–101.

[41] Review article: Reproduction in the patient with inflammatory bowel disease. Heetun ZS, Byrnes C, Neary P, O'Morain C. *Aliment Pharmacol Ther*. 2007 Aug 15;26(4):513-33.

[42] Blanford AT, Murphy BE. In vitro metabolism of prednisolone, dexamethasone, betamethasone, and cortisol by the human placenta. *Am J Obstet Gynecol* 1977; 127: 264–7.

[43] Dancis J, Jansen V, Levitz M. Placental transfer of steroids: effect of binding to serum albumin and to placenta. *Am J Physiol* 1980;238: E208–13.

[44] Milunsky A, Graef JW, Gaynor MF Jr. Methotrexate-induced congenital malformations. *J Pediatr* 1968; 72: 790–5.

[45] De Boer NK, Jarbandhan SV, De Graaf P, Mulder CJ, Van Elburg RM, Van Bodegraven AA. Azathioprine use during pregnancy: unexpected intrauterine exposure to metabolites. *Am J Gastroenterol* 2006; 101: 1390–2.

[46] Janssen NM, Genta MS. The effects of immunosuppressive and anti-inflammatory medications on fertility, pregnancy, and lactation. *Arch Intern Med* 2000; 160: 610–9.

[47] Davison JM, Dellagrammatikas H, Parkin JM. Maternal azathioprine therapy and depressed haemopoiesis in the babies of renal allograft patients. *Br J Obstet Gynecol* 1985; 92: 233–9.

[48] Norgard B, Pedersen L, Fonager K, Rasmussen SN, Sorensen HT. Azathioprine, mercaptopurine and birth outcome: a population-based cohort study. *Aliment Pharmacol Ther* 2003; 17: 827–34.

[49] Alstead EM, Ritchie JK, Lennard-Jones JE, Farthing MJ, Clark ML. Safety of azathioprine in pregnancy in inflammatory bowel disease. *Gastroenterology* 1990; 99: 443–6.

[50] Oefferlbauer-Ernst A, Reinisch W, Miehsler W, Vogelsang H, Dejaco C. Healthy offspring in parents both receiving thiopurines. *Gastroenterology* 2004; 126: 628.

[51] Shim L, Eslick GD, Simring AA, Murray H, Weltman MD.The effects of azathioprine on birth outcomes in women with inflammatory bowel disease (IBD). *J Crohns Colitis*. 2011 Jun;5(3):234-8.

[52] Coelho J, et al. Pregnancy outcome in patients with inflammatory bowel disease treated with thiopurines: cohort from the CESAME Study.; CESAME Pregnancy Study Group (France). *Gut*. 2011 Feb;60(2):198-203.

[53] Albengres E, Le Louet H, Tillement JP. Immunosuppressive drugs and pregnancy: experimental and clinical data. *Transplant Proc*1997; 29: 2461–6.

[54] Mason RJ, Thomson AW, Whiting PH, et al. Cyclosporine-induced fetotoxicity in the rat. *Transplantation* 1985;39:9-12.

[55] Bar Oz B, Hackman R, Einarson T, Koren G. Pregnancy outcome after cyclosporine therapy during pregnancy: a meta-analysis. *Transplantation*. 2001 Apr 27;71(8):1051-5.

[56] Anderson JB, Turner GM, Williamson RC. Fulminant ulcerative colitis in late pregnancy and the puerperium. *J R Soc Med* 1987;80: 492–4.
[57] Zelinkova Z, et al. High intra-uterine exposure to infliximab following maternal anti-TNF treatment during pregnancy. *Aliment Pharmacol Ther.* 2011 May;33(9):1053-8.
[58] Schnitzler F, et al. Outcome of pregnancy in women with inflammatory bowel disease treated with antitumor necrosis factor therapy. *Inflamm Bowel Dis.* 2011 Jan 6. [Epub ahead of print].
[59] Cheent K et al Case Report: Fatal case of disseminated BCG infection in an infant born to a mother taking infliximab for Crohn's disease. *J Crohns Colitis.* 2010 Nov;4(5):603-5.
[60] Sorensen HT, Larsen H, Jensen ES, et al. Safety of metronidazole during pregnancy: a cohort study of risk of congenital abnormalities, preterm delivery and low birth weight in 124 women. *J Antimicrob Chemother* 1999; 44: 854–6.
[61] Diav-Citrin O, Shechtman S, Gotteiner T, Arnon J, Ornoy A. Pregnancy outcome after gestational exposure to metronidazole: a prospective controlled cohort study. *Teratology* 2001; 63: 186–92.
[62] Loebstein R, Addis A, Ho E, et al. Pregnancy outcome following gestational exposure to fluoroquinolones: a multicenter prospective controlled study. *Antimicrob Agents Chemother* 1998; 42: 1336–9.
[63] Einarson A, Mastroiacovo P, Arnon J, et al. Prospective, controlled, multicentre study of loperamide in pregnancy. *Can J Gastroenterol* 2000; 14: 185–7.
[64] Kallen B, Nilsson E, Olausson PO. Maternal use of loperamide in early pregnancy and delivery outcomes. *Acta Paediatrica* 2008;97:541-5.
[65] Bergstrand O, Hellers G. Breast-feeding during infancy in patients who later develop Crohn's disease. *Scand J Gastroenterol* 1983; 18: 903–6.
[66] Kane S, Lemieux N. The role of breastfeeding in postpartum disease activity in women with inflammatory bowel disease. *Am J Gastroenterol* 2005; 100: 102–5.
[67] Silverman DA, Ford J, Shaw I, Probert CS. Is mesalazine really safe for use in breastfeeding mothers? *Gut* 2005; 54: 170–1.
[68] Branski D, Kerem E, Gross-Kieselstein E, Hurvitz H, Litt R, Abrahamov A. Bloody diarrhea - a possible complication of sulfasalazine transferred through human breast milk. *J Pediatr Gastroenterol Nutr* 1986; 5: 316–7.
[69] Nelis G. Diarrhoea due to 5-aminosalicylic acid in breast milk. *Lancet* 1989; i: 383.
[70] Ferrero S, Ragni N. Inflammatory bowel disease: management issues during pregnancy. *Arch Gynaecol Obstet* 2004; 270: 79–85.
[71] Jusko WJ. Pharmacokinetics and receptor-mediated pharmacodynamics of corticosteroids. *Toxicology* 1995; 102: 189–96.
[72] Angelberger S, et al. Long term follow-up of babies exposed to azathioprine in utero and b=via breast feeding. *J Crohns Coliltis*, 2011. Apr;5(2):95-100.
[73] Committee on Drugs American Academy of Pediatrics. Transfer of drugs and other chemicals into human milk. *Pediatrics* 2001; 108: 776–9.
[74] Kane et al. Absence of infliximab in infants and breast milk from nursing mothers receiving therapy for Crohn's disease before and after delivery. *J Clin Gastroenterol.* 2009; 43: 613-616.

[75] Mahadevan U, Kane S. American Gastroenterological Association Institute Technical Review on the use of gastrointestinal medications in pregnancy. *Gastroenterology* 2006; 131: 283–311.

[76] Gert Van Assche, Axel Digness, Walter Reinisch, et al. The second European evidence-based consensus on the diagnosis and management of Crohn's Disease: special situations. *Journal of Crohn's and Colitis* (2010)4,63-101.

9

Ulcerative Colitis in Children and Adolescents

Andrew S. Day[1,2,3] and Daniel A. Lemberg[2,3]
[1]*Department of Paediatrics, University of Otago (Christchurch), Christchurch,*
[2]*School of Women's and Children's Health, University of New South Wales,*
[3]*Department of Gastroenterology, Sydney Children's Hospital, Randwick, Sydney, NSW,*
[1]*New Zealand*
[2,3]*Australia*

1. Introduction

Ulcerative colitis (UC) is a chronic gastrointestinal inflammatory disorder and is one of the inflammatory bowel diseases (IBD) along with Crohn disease (CD). CD can involve any area of the gastrointestinal (GI) tract and has features of transmural disease, skip lesions and mucosal granulomata. UC, on the other hand, principally involves the colon for a variable length, and comprises confluent superficial inflammation. In addition, some individuals may be termed to have IBD unclassified (IBDU): a situation where there are clear diagnostic features of IBD, but no definitive features of either UC or CD. Over time many individuals with IBDU are reclassified as UC or CD. At present CD and UC are considered to be incurable, although colectomy can be seen as a surgical cure for UC. Furthermore, the pathogenesis of these conditions remains unclear, although understanding is increasing rapidly.

The onset of UC can be in any age, from the first year of life. The peak age of onset, however, is between 15 and 35 years of age. Overall rates of UC climbed through the last decades of the 20th century. Recent paediatric data suggests that rates of UC have been static in a number of countries. In some, however, UC incidence has continued to increase. In countries where IBD was previously uncommon, UC incidence rates are also noted to be increasingly recently. When diagnosed in children of any age, these individuals face a long-term condition with remitting-relapsing features. Children may have significant interruption to daily activities and consequent impact upon quality of life (QOL). A number will have complications of disease and some will require colectomy during childhood. Because of the multiple aspects of UC and the various adverse impacts, children and adolescents with UC should be considered separately to adults with UC and require a multidisciplinary approach to management to ensure that all aspects are considered in optimal fashion.

2. Pathogenesis of IBD

2.1 Current hypothesis of causation of UC

At the present the precise cause of IBD is unknown. The best accepted hypothesis is that UC develops in individuals at genetic risk as a result of interactions between the intestinal microflora and the host innate immune responses, leading to dysregulated immune responses and to consequent inflammation. Environmental factors are also important.

2.2 Genetic influences in the development of UC

The familial nature of UC and of CD has been recognised for many years. Over the last decade or so, international collaborative groups have focused on identifying the genetic elements contributing to the risk of IBD, with many key discoveries. Over 100 loci are now reported in association with IBD. There is some overlap with many loci important for both CD and UC. However, more than 20 loci are specific for UC. These include genes encoding for cytokines (e.g. interleukin (IL)-10, IL-22 and IL-26) and others whose function are unclear (e.g. ARPC2) (Thompson and Lees 2011; Cho and Brant 2011).

Recent studies have used genome wide association studies (GWAS) to examine particular genetic elements important in early-onset (paediatric) UC and have demonstrated the involvement of several particular genes (Anderson et al 2011; Henderson et al 2011a). Important mutations have been shown in IL-27 (implicated in Th17 cell function), CAPN10 (involved in endoplasmic reticulum stress responses), MTMR3 (component of autophagy reactions), and several other genes.

2.3 The intestinal flora and UC

The intestinal flora is clearly critical in the development of IBD. In specific animal models of gut inflammation, exclusion of the bacterial flora prevents or delays the onset of the inflammatory changes. In the human setting, excluding the flow of faecal effluent from an involved segment of bowel (i.e. defunctioning a segment of the bowel) leads to improvement of inflammation. Furthermore, antibiotic treatment of individuals with active CD can lead to improvement, whilst probiotic therapies that modify the intestinal flora have similar effects in the setting of UC.

At present, however, there is no evidence for one specific organism or group of organisms being the causative agent(s) of IBD. Candidate organisms include *Mycobacterium paratuberculosis* (MAP), *Escherichia coli*, and mucous-associated flora. Recent work has focused on several mucous-associated flora and indicates high rates of specific organisms in children with active IBD compared to controls. *Campylobacter concisus* is one example of a bacterium that may play roles in the development of IBD. Our work in Australian children has illustrated that this organism is frequently present at the time of diagnosis of CD in children (Man et al 2010). Ongoing studies from the UK also indicate that this organism is more often present in newly diagnosed UC than in controls (Mukhopadhya et al 2011). However, at present there is not sufficient data to indicate that this pathogen is the specific causative agent in IBD.

2.4 Other environmental factors

Other environmental factors are also relevant to the development of UC. Appendectomy for appendicitis is associated with lower rates of UC, whilst smoking also can be protective (Bastida et al 2011). Exposure to second-hand smoke (passive smoking) in children does not appear to provide any protection against the development of UC (Mahid et al 2007). However, one series suggested that patients with UC exposed to passive smoke had increased extra-intestinal manifestations (van der Heide 2011), but this has not been described by others. Other factors that are shown to be protective against UC include having a vegetable garden as a child and breast-feeding (Gearry et al 2010).

2.5 Dysregulated immune responses

Disrupted innate defence mechanisms in the gut are also critical to the development of the chronic inflammation as seen in IBD. Many of the genes implicated in IBD encode for proteins involved in innate protection of the mucosa. Altered barrier function, leading to increased epithelial permeability, is clearly described. It is unclear if this is a primary event, or if it occurs secondary to gut inflammation. Variation in innate antibacterial proteins, such as defensins, may contribute to altered host responses (Ramasundara et al 2009). Altered immune responses are likely also important. T helper cell type 1 (Th1) responses have traditionally been implicated in CD, whilst Th2 or a combination of both pathways seen as relevant to UC. More recent understanding suggests that T regulatory cells (Tregs) have key roles in UC.

3. Epidemiology of UC in children and adolescents

UC can occur in children of any age, but rates tend to increase with age. Most large cohorts illustrate that UC comprises around 25-30% of paediatric IBD (the majority of children with IBD are diagnosed with CD). Family history of IBD (CD or UC) is commonly seen in children diagnosed with UC.

Two large cohorts have examined the epidemiology of paediatric UC in different areas of the USA. The earlier study retrospectively reviewed 171 children diagnosed with UC in two academic centres in North-East USA (Hyams et al 1996). The children in the cohort ranged from the second year of life to almost 18 years of age (mean 11.7 yrs). Just over one third of the group were aged less than 10 years at diagnosis. The gender distribution slightly favoured males (55%) and the population was predominantly Caucasian (95%). A first degree family history was present in 11%. Most had symptoms for less than 3 months, but 18% had symptoms for more than 6 months duration before diagnosis. At diagnosis, mild disease was present in 43%, with moderate or severe disease in 57%. The majority of the mild group had proctitis or proctosigmoiditis, whilst almost the entire moderate/severe group had left-sided or pan-colonic disease. Ninety percent of the mild group and 80% of the mod/severe group had cessation of symptoms within the first six months of therapy. Almost two thirds of the mild group had inactive disease in the second six-month period after diagnosis, with only one child having continuous disease in this time period. Over the same period, 11% of the moderate/severe group had continuous disease, with a further 44% having intermittent/chronic disease course. Disease distribution did not appear to influence this course. Twenty-seven percent of the mild group received corticosteroids by 12 months after diagnosis, contrasting with 70% of the moderate/severe group needing this therapy over the same time. Overall, the one year colectomy rate in this group of children was 9% at 12 months and 19% at 5 years. Age less than 10 years did not influence colectomy rates, but initial disease severity was associated with increased risk for colectomy overall.

More recently was a study of prospectively recruited children with diagnosis of IBD from across the state of Wisconsin for the first two years of the 21st century (Kugathasan et al 2003). Sixty children with UC were identified within a total of 199 children with IBD (30% of the total). The UC cohort had an average age of 11.8 yrs and 55% were male. There was no association between UC and rural or urban location and 87% were Caucasian. Eleven percent had a first or second-degree family member with IBD. Ninety-eight percent of this group had diarrhoea at diagnosis, with bleeding in 83%, pain in 43% and weight loss in 38%.

The mean period of symptoms prior to diagnosis was 3 months in this group. Most of the group (90%) had pan-colonic disease, with the rest having left-sided location. ESR was normal in 35% and albumin was normal in 68% of the cohort.

Follow-up data including response to therapy, or other outcomes were not reported in this cohort.

A recent report examined the incidence of UC across Scotland in two distinct time periods (1990-95 and 2003-8) (Henderson et al 2011b). Compared to the earlier time period, the incidence was greater in the more recent cohort (1.59/100,000/yr versus 2.06/100,000/yr; p=0.023). This equates to a 30% increase in paediatric UC over this period. There was a male predominance overall and age-adjusted incidence figures showed increases in males but not females over time. Another recent study utilised Canadian health data and demonstrated a modest rise on the prevalence of UC from 16.2 to 19.7/100,000 over the period of 1994 to 2005 (Benchimol et al 2009).

The overall trends in the rates of UC were reviewed recently (Benchimol et al 2011). This article assessed 139 studies reporting rates of paediatric-onset IBD across 32 countries, both developing and developed. Overall, rates of IBD were clearly shown to be increasing with varied rates between countries. Not all the studies applied statistical analysis to changing rates over time: overall one-fifth of the studies showed increasing UC in children.

A recent report has characterised patterns of UC in Japanese children with direct comparison to adults in that country (Ishige et al 2010). A long-standing register was examined for the patterns of disease in children and adults. In total, 37,846 individuals with UC were included: 5.9% were aged less than 16 years of age. The children more commonly had positive first-degree family history, more severe disease at diagnosis and had more extensive colitis than adults. Family history of IBD was seen in 4.3% of the children (less than in comparable European cohorts).

Reports from the middle part of the 20th century illustrate a predominance of UC in cohorts of IBD. As noted above, most recent cohorts reported in the western world demonstrate much higher rates of CD than UC. One study has however, demonstrated that this is not a universal change (Lehtinen et al 2011). This study of rates of paediatric IBD in Finland over 16 years showed increasing rates of IBD over this time (rates increased by 6.5% per annum. In addition, rates of UC increased from 4/100,000 to 9/100,000 over the period from 1992 to 2003. These regional differences illustrate the importance of environmental factors in the development of UC.

Interestingly, recent reports from Asia, where IBD was previously considered to be rare, have shown increasing rates of UC (more so than with CD) (Goh and Xiao 2009). This pattern of differing rates across the globe also illustrates the importance of environmental factors.

4. Phenotypic features of UC

UC has traditionally been seen as a chronic inflammatory condition of the colon, with inflammation extending for variable distances from the anus. Disease patterns include proctitis (distal changes only), left-sided colitis or pan-colitis.

Inflammation is superficial, with acute and chronic changes. This pattern contrasts with CD, where disease can involve any section of the gastrointestinal tract (from mouth to anus), with trans-mural inflammatory changes and the presence of the specific findings of granulomas. Perianal disease is a feature of CD and not UC.

The adult-based Montreal disease classification system for IBD included three types of UC: proctitis (E1), left-sided disease (E2) or disease proximal to the splenic flexure (E3) (Silverberg et al 2005). The recent Paris classification has adjusted the Montreal system for paediatric UC by the addition of E4 (disease proximal to hepatic flexure), and S1 (ever severe UC) (Levine et al 2011).

Recent studies demonstrate that non-specific gastritis may be seen in combination with colonic disease in UC (Hori et al 2008). Homing of lymphocytes from the colon to the stomach may explain some of these events (Berrebi et al 2003). In addition some authors describe so-called "back-wash" ileitis, with minor changes present in the distal ileum, as an occasional feature of UC.

UC is associated with various extra-intestinal manifestations (EIM) of disease, such as skin, eye and liver disease. EIM were noted in 285 of a cohort of 1009 newly diagnosed patients with IBD - most of these occurred within the first 12 months after diagnosis (Dotson et al 2011). In a cohort of 211 children with UC from the UK, 1 had skin manifestations and 5 had liver disease at diagnosis (Sawczenko et al 2003).

Several studies of large paediatric cohorts have illustrated key phenotypic features of UC. These studies demonstrate that many children have pan-colitis at diagnosis, with few having proctitis and a small number having left-sided disease. Furthermore, many children with limited disease at initial assessment have extension to pan-colonic disease over the first 2-3 years of their disease. This pattern in children contrasts greatly with adult UC, where proctitis is prominent and pan-colitis seen less commonly.

A study based in Scotland evaluated the features of 99 children with UC at diagnosis and over the subsequent years, and compared these features of a cohort of adult-onset UC (Van Limbergen et al 2008). UC was extensive (pan-colonic) in 82% of the children at the time of diagnosis. In contrast, this pattern was seen in just 48% of adults ($p < 0.0001$). Almost half (46%) of the children without extensive disease initially progressed to develop extensive colitis during follow-up. One third of the group required immunomodulatory therapy within 12 months of diagnosis. In addition, the median time to first surgery was substantially shorter in the patients with childhood-onset than in adult-onset patients.

A similar cohort was described from France, in which 112 children were characterised at diagnosis and their progress followed for at least 2 years (Gower-Rosseau et al 2009). At diagnosis, 28% of the children had proctitis, 35% left-sided colitis, and 37% extensive colitis. The disease course of this group also was characterized by disease extension in 49% of patients. Delay in diagnosis for more than 6 months and a positive family history of IBD were associated with an increased risk of extension of disease. Eight percent of this group had colectomy within 12 months of diagnosis. By 3 years, 15% had colectomy and by 5 years 20% had undergone colectomy. The risk of colectomy was increased if EIM were present at diagnosis (hazard ratio = 3.5 (1.2-10.5)). In addition, with regards the group with less extensive disease initially, those who had disease progression had much greater risk of needing colectomy than those who continued to have restricted disease. These two well-described cohorts of children from Europe have illustrated a number of key aspects of the natural history and outcomes of paediatric UC, and have emphasised that paediatric-onset disease has many key differences from the same disease beginning in adulthood.

5. Presentation patterns of UC

Bloody diarrhoea is the most common presenting feature in paediatric UC. However, children may also have less specific symptoms of abdominal pain, anaemia, or lethargy.

In a large cohort of British children (n=172) newly diagnosed with UC, diarrhoea was seen in 72%, bleeding in 84%, pain in 62%, weight loss in 31%, and lethargy in 12% (Sawczenko et al 2003). Arthropathy, nausea and secondary amenorrhoea were seen less commonly.

Idiopathic acute pancreatitis (AP) is a further atypical pattern of presentation with UC. Broide et al (Broide et al 2011) retrospectively evaluated a cohort of 12 individuals with IBD who had presented initially with AP: 10 of these were children. Eight of these 10 children had colonic disease (four with UC). Although the median time between the episode of AP and the onset of IBD was 24 weeks, the longest duration was 156 weeks.

Acute severe UC (or fulminant colitis) can be seen at diagnosis or at subsequent exacerbations in adults or children with UC. In adults this pattern is defined as more than six bloody motions daily along with tachycardia, fever, anaemia or elevated ESR (one of these required for the definition). In children acute severe colitis can be defined as Pediatric Ulcerative colitis activity index (PUCAI) of 65 points or greater.

Historically, acute severe colitis was seen as a medical emergency with a high case fatality rate. It remains a life-threatening condition, with risk of various complications. Hence early recognition and optimal management of this condition is critical.

6. Growth and nutrition in paediatric UC

Children with UC commonly have weight loss at presentation. Case series suggest that up to 65% of children with UC have a history of weight loss at diagnosis (Griffiths et al 2004). In addition to weight loss and/or failure to continue gaining weight normally, children diagnosed with UC may also have a history of interrupted or impaired linear growth. As many children with UC are diagnosed in adolescence, before or during their pubertal growth spurt, perturbation of normal linear growth at the time of the expected pubertal growth spurt can be a significant complication of paediatric IBD. For these reasons, ongoing attention to growth and nutrition from the time of diagnosis and thereafter, is a crucial aspect of management of UC in children and adolescents. These concerns, however, are even more pertinent in children with CD, which has much greater impact on growth and nutrition than in paediatric UC.

6.1 Overweight and obesity in IBD

Although most concern about the nutritional impact of IBD in children is with regards under nutrition, recent data indicates that more children are overweight (BMI > 85%) and/or obese (BMI > 95%) at the time of diagnosis of IBD. These changes may simply reflect recent overall changes in weight in children and adolescents across many countries (i.e. increasing overweight/obesity). However, overweight/obese status has important implications for children with IBD.

In a group of 166 children with newly diagnosed IBD in Wisconsin, USA, 17.6% of the children with UC were overweight/obese (Sondike et al 2004). More recently, 23.3% of a separate group of 1598 American children with known CD and UC were noted to be overweight/obese (Long et al 2011). The rate of over nutrition was markedly greater (30%) in the children with UC in this group than the children with CD. In this cohort recruited from a number of paediatric centres, overweight/obesity status was associated with African-American ethnicity and Medicaid insurance. In addition, prior surgical intervention was linked with overweight/obese status in the children with CD, suggesting that the presence of over nutrition may be associated with a more severe disease course. Overweight/obese status may also make medical therapies more difficult, and increase surgical morbidities. In addition, it may increase psychological outcomes in the setting of children with a chronic disease, making them stand out even more from their peers.

7. Investigation and diagnosis of UC in children and adolescents

7.1 Consideration of diagnosis of IBD

The diagnosis of UC relies firstly upon consideration of the diagnosis. Children with atypical symptoms may be reassured and symptoms not assessed further if practitioners are not aware that UC can present at any age. As noted above, presentation patterns in children with UC vary, with most typical symptoms being bleeding, diarrhoea and pain. Family history of IBD (especially in first degree family members) should further raise suspicion of possible IBD.

A presentation with bloody diarrhoea in a child requires a series of assessments. In infants, the differential of this presentation includes eosinophilic (allergic) colitis, infection, surgical conditions (such as intussusception) and complications of congenital conditions (such as Meckels diverticulum). In older children, infection is an important differential. Functional constipation with bleeding from distal causes (anal fissures) and perianal Streptococcal infection may be important to exclude.

7.2 Approach to possible IBD/UC

A detailed history should clarify the features of the gastrointestinal symptoms, especially patterns of pain and bowel habit. Appetite, energy levels (lethargy), and weight changes should be documented clearly. The presence of any extra-intestinal features should be detailed, including skin, eyes, joint and systemic symptoms. Past history of gastrointestinal symptoms and diseases should be noted, along with family history of IBD or other GI conditions. The extent to which the child has been able to continue daily activities should be carefully documented also: this includes attendance at school, school performance, social interactions, ability to undertake sports or other hobbies, and general interest in these activities. Clarification of current immunisations status is important and a catch-up plan arranged if required. Confirmation of past history of varicella or of antibody protection against this infection will be relevant if this vaccine is not included in the routine schedule.

Physical examination should include a search for extra-intestinal manifestations of IBD (skin for erythema nodosum or pyoderma gangrenosum, joints for arthalgia/arthritis and mouth for ulceration or lip swelling), documentation of oedema, anaemia and clubbing, and comprehensive examination of abdomen and perianal region. The abdomen should be examined for signs of organomegaly, tenderness and mass. Perianal region should be examined for signs of skin tags, fissures, fistulas or collections. Examination of lower spine and ileo-sacral region may be relevant if back pain is a feature.

In addition, to these undertakings a close examination of growth and nutrition is also relevant. This should begin with detailed examination for nutritional deficiencies, such as anaemia, oedema and skin changes. Current weight and height measurements should be recorded and plotted on a standard age-appropriate growth chart. BMI should be calculated. Retrieval of past weight and height measurements is often helpful to fully document the child's growth history and patterns over time. These measurements can be used to calculate recent height velocity. Parental and family growth patterns are also important to define. In peri-pubertal children Tanner stage should be documented to clearly define current pubertal status. Establishment of the child's current bone age (using radiograph of the child's left wrist) will be helpful in interpreting any linear growth delay.

7.3 Initial investigations

The first investigations in the setting of possible UC include the collection of multiple stool samples for microscopy and culture to exclude enteric infection. Testing should include the request for specific organisms including *Clostridium difficile.* Further tests should include blood tests for serum markers of inflammation (as per below section), and stool inflammatory markers (see below section) if available.

Other tests may be indicated in the initial work-up depending on the clinical context - two further examples are investigations for possible Coeliac disease (tissue transglutaminase and total immunoglobulin A) and tests for pancreatitis (amylase and lipase).

If infection is excluded and the results of initial tests indicate inflammatory events, then endoscopic assessment should next be undertaken. International guidelines recommend colonoscopy (with terminal ileal intubation) and upper gastrointestinal endoscopy for the assessment of possible IBD in children. Multiple biopsies from all segments of the upper and lower gut are required to ensure full assessment of the GI tract.

Assessment of the small bowel is also required to exclude the presence of small bowel CD and to distinguish from UC. The preferred test in many centres is now small bowel magnetic resonance imaging (MRI), known either as MRI enterography or small bowel series MRI. This modality has better sensitivity and specificity than some other modalities that been used in the past, such as barium meal and follow-through or technetium-labelled white cell scan. Capsule endoscopy and positron-emission tomography (PET scanning) also have high test utility, but remain less available or more expensive options at present.

7.4 Further baseline assessment after confirmation of UC

Other baseline testing should include assessment of renal function (serum urea and creatinine), liver chemistry (Bilirubin, ALT, AST, GGT, ALP and albumin), electrolytes and minerals (sodium, potassium, chloride, calcium, phosphate, magnesium and zinc), and nutritional or absorptive markers (iron, ferritin, vitamin B12, folate and Vitamin D).

Serological markers may be helpful in differentiating between CD and UC if these are available. The presence of anti-neutrophil cytoplasmic antibodies (p-ANCA) is more common in UC, whereas anti-*Saccharomyces cerevisiae* antibodies (ASCA) are more frequently found in CD.

It also may be appropriate to define TPMT activity at the time of baseline assessment, so that this result is available in the event of future prescription of thiopurines.

7.5 Endoscopic and histologic features of UC

The typical endoscopic appearance in UC is of confluent disease extending proximally from the rectum for a variable distance. Ulcers, erythema, loss of normal vascular pattern, granularity, increased friability and the presence of pseudopolyps are common findings (**Figure 1**). An absence of skip lesions is one aspect to assist in excluding CD. Although rectal sparing is typically seen as a feature of CD, some authors have suggested that this may be present in UC (Rajwal et al 2004).

Histologically, typical changes of UC include a continuous pattern of acute and chronic mucosal inflammation, with crypt distortion, crypt abscesses, and goblet cell depletion. The absence of granulomas or of patchy changes helps to exclude from CD.

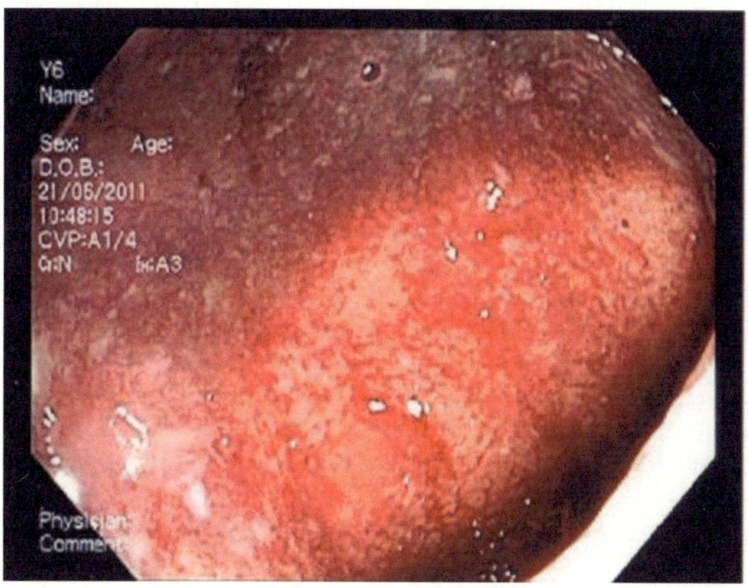

Fig. 1. Typical endoscopic appearance of severe colitis, with loss of normal mucosal vascular patterns, oedema, friability and ulceration

7.6 Radiologic findings in UC

As mentioned above, examination of the small bowel should be included as an essential part of the work-up for likely IBD. The principal rationale is to define the extent or presence of small bowel CD, which may not be evident on standard endoscopic assessment. In UC, the small bowel radiology assessment would be expected to be normal.

Plain abdominal radiographs may show changes of colitis in UC, with thumb-printing, wall thickening or featureless mucosal surface. Plain radiographs should also be considered in the assessment of fulminant (acute severe) colitis where abdominal tenderness or distension is present to ascertain if toxic megacolon is present. Abdominal ultrasound may also be used to define colonic wall thickening and due to improved sensitivity is being considered more.

In the event of incomplete colonoscopy (such as in the settings of colonic stricture or very severe mucosal disease), imaging may be helpful to confirm the proximal extent of the colonic involvement. Magnetic resonance imaging or labelled white cell scans may be helpful. Barium enema examinations can be considered if other tests are not feasible or are unhelpful, but are no longer first-line investigations in children.

7.7 Differentiation between CD and UC

A full assessment is important to definitively establish a diagnosis of IBD and also to assist in distinguishing between UC and CD. Almost two thirds of children with CD have upper gut and/or small bowel changes at diagnosis. These may be the only locations of disease, or may help to delineate the diagnosis in the setting of pan-colitis where there are no other defining features of UC or CD present.

The European Society for Paediatric Gastroenterology, Hepatology and Nutrition (ESPGHAN) established the Porto criteria in 2005 (ESPGHAN 2005). This consensus statement provided a set of recommendations for the key elements for the diagnosis of IBD and also considered the important features to distinguish between CD and UC. A Spanish group has subsequently reviewed a cohort of 108 patients according to the application of the Porto criteria (Martin De Carpi et al 2011). Overall they noted that these criteria had been followed in 49% of the children (with a higher percentage after the publication of the criteria than prior to this). Ileocolonoscopy was undertaken in 85.2% of children with multiple biopsies obtained. Upper endoscopy was undertaken in 39% of children prior to and 72% of the group after the publication of the Porto criteria. These authors noted that the introduction of the criteria lead to a change in clinical practice.

A report from a NASPGHAN working group considered the key elements in differentiating between UC and CD in children or adolescents (NASPGHAN 2007). This report aimed to address controversies in the assessment of IBD in children and to develop an algorithm to enhance practitioner agreement and consistency in the diagnosis and classification of CD and UC. Clarification of the features of IBD-Unclassified (IBDU) was also undertaken.

8. Inflammatory markers and disease activity in paediatric UC

8.1 Assessment of disease activity: Pediatric UC Activity Index

Recently the Pediatric UC activity index (PUCAI) has been developed as a standardised measure of activity in children with UC (Turner et al 2007). A well-defined process was used to identify six critical elements (from an initial group of 41 variables). These six variables are abdominal pain, rectal bleeding, stool consistency, nocturnal stools, number of stools each 24 hours and interruption to normal activities. The PUCAI correlates closely with other indicators, such as physician global assessment and endoscopic scores (Turner et al 2009). This validated score, which is simple and non-invasive, can now be used to assess disease activity and to monitor changes in activity following intervention. It can also be used to guide management decisions, such as in the context of acute severe UC.

8.2 Relapse and remission in paediatric UC

UC tends to follow a relapsing and remitting course, with periods of disease control interrupted by relapses or flares of symptoms. Active disease in children with UC can be defined in terms of symptoms, serum or faecal markers of inflammation and increased mucosal inflammatory changes. In contrast, remission in children can be defined clinically or symptomatically (resolution of symptoms), biochemically (normalisation of abnormal inflammatory markers) and histologically (mucosal healing). Mucosal healing is increasingly recognised as an important goal in the initial management of IBD, especially in children with many years of disease ahead of them. Attaining mucosal healing may in turn lead to modification of the long-term disease course in UC (Colombel et al, 2011). Although mucosal healing is now seen as an ideal state, in terms of long-term outcomes, this degree of monitoring requires repeated endoscopic and colonoscopic assessment, which is often not feasible or possible in children.

8.3 Standard serum inflammatory markers

Standard serum markers of inflammation include ESR, CRP, platelets and albumin. These markers are easy to measure in most routine clinical laboratories, but tend to have low specificity and sensitivity for gut inflammation in children with UC. Mack et al measured ESR, platelet count, albumin level along with haemoglobin in 134 children with newly diagnosed UC (Mack et al 2007). All four of these markers were normal in 54% of the children with mild UC, whilst 4.3% of those with moderate-severe UC had normal tests. ESR was the most useful test in this cohort. In addition, disease extent was linked with the number of abnormal tests.

In a small cohort of 30 children with diagnosed with UC at Sydney Children's Hospital (Sydney, Australia), 54% had elevated ESR, whilst platelets were elevated in 13%, CRP high in 29% and albumin abnormal in 33% (Day et al, unpublished data). There was no correlation between disease location and the number of abnormal results in this group.

In a further, recently reported, cohort of 102 Canadian children with newly diagnosed UC, CRP levels were found to be elevated in 41% of those with mild disease and 60% of those with moderate-severe disease (Tsampalieros et al 2011).

8.4 Faecal markers of inflammation

Stool samples can be used to measure various markers of gut inflammation. The presence of faecal white cells can indicate the presence of gut inflammation but are also present in various enteric infections. Faecal white blood cells may be degraded if the sample is not viewed promptly. Elevated levels of faecal α-1-antitrypsin, a protein that is stable in stool, can reflect mucosal inflammation as a breach of the epithelium may lead to a protein losing state. Neither of these indicators has adequate sensitivity and specificity.

Other faecal markers of inflammation include calprotectin, S100A12, and lactoferrin. Although these three markers are not yet universally available, they provide a less-invasive method to assess gut inflammation. Normalisation of these markers can be used as markers of the success of therapy. Each of the measures can be used to assess the response to therapeutic intervention in children with UC. Calprotectin can also be helpful in assessing the risk of subsequent relapse of disease (Costa et al 2005).

9. Principles of management of UC in children

The overall aims of management of UC in children and adolescents are to control inflammation and to maintain remission, whilst ensuring that the child has normal growth and development. Ongoing inflammation will likely adversely impact upon growth in children and adolescents.

As well as optimising growth, management should ensure normal pubertal development, and normal social and psychological health. Treatment side-effects must be avoided or minimised: especially those side-effects that may in turn interfere with growth and development. Thus, therapeutic choices must be seen in the context not just of the child's current disease status and disease location, but also in terms of growth, puberty, bone health, family setting, and psychological wellbeing. In addition to the critical importance of growth and nutrition in children, it is also crucial to ensure the avoidance of side effects in children who will face many years of disease and exposure to medications. One other element of the long term nature of these diseases, when commencing in childhood, is that reduction and control of the disease burden may help to avoid long-term disease related complications. One example of this is the increased risk of colonic cancer seen in the setting of long-standing colitis (colitis associated carcinoma), especially when uncontrolled.

Due to the complex medical and social issues involved in the management and treatment of children and adolescents with CD or UC, care should be provided in a multi-disciplinary manner. In addition to the management of medical aspects by specialist paediatric gastroenterologists, universal attention must be paid to many other issues. These include growth and nutrition, normal development, attention to schooling and learning, psychosocial issues, coping and adjustment issues, and general well-being. In addition to the various direct effects of chronic UC upon the child or adolescent patient, these chronic illnesses may also impact adversely upon siblings and parents.

These wide ranging and important issues mean that many key non-medical personnel also should be closely involved in the care of these children. These individuals include nursing staff (to provide key liaison and coordination roles), dietitians (growth and nutrition), social workers and psychologists (psychosocial and coping aspects). Paediatric surgeons, pathologists and radiologists experienced and skilled in relevant aspects of paediatric UC also comprise key personnel contributing to the care of children with UC. The child's general practitioner also plays an important role in the care of these children. Thus the management of all children with CD or UC should be facilitated within a context that provides access to each of these professionals. The system of care needs to be able to provide coordination of services, with good clear lines of communication between personnel.

Further to the personnel requirements for an environment caring for children with CD and UC, appropriate support is also necessary. This includes adequate administration support (such as secretarial, outpatient booking staff and medical record staff), along with adequate record and database systems. This may include systems to ensure regular checking of required blood tests, or annual blood tests, or providing for clear records of complications or events. This might include the use of diagnostic checklists, pre-clinic review meetings, proformas for clinic review and systems to ensure regular monitoring requirements. These database and record keeping resources will provide for smooth seamless clinical management, and also for eventual transition to adult services and audit or research activities.

A further key principle in the management of children with UC is that care needs to be firmly family focused. A child with UC needs to be seen in the context of their family. Parents and sometimes siblings will attend outpatient appointments with their child. Parents and the patient will be together involved in decision making or consideration of therapeutic choices. Furthermore, parents and the patient's siblings will be directly and indirectly affected by the child's condition.

10. Medical management of paediatric UC

10.1 Induction and maintenance of remission in UC

The therapies proven to have roles in the induction of remission of active UC in children are less numerous than those available for CD. Overall therapies can be considered as those used to induce remission and those used to maintain remission (**Table 1**).

INDUCE REMISSION	MAINTAIN REMISSION
Corticosteroids	Corticosteroids (especially topical)
ASA	ASA
Tacrolimus (or cyclosporin)	Azathioprine / 6-mercaptopurine
Infliximab	Methotrexate
?Adalimumab	?Tacrolimus
	?Infliximab

Table 1. Standard Therapies for UC in children and adolescents

As in CD, the goal in the long term management of UC in children is to maintain remission and control of disease, along with ensuring optimisation of normal life events, whilst ensuring that medical therapy does not lead to adverse consequences.

CS are most commonly used to induce remission, although ASA may have a role in mild disease. Tacrolimus, cyclosporin and infliximab may have roles in severe UC, as second line (rescue) therapy. Two therapies that have roles in paediatric CD (exclusive enteral nutrition and antibiotics) probably do not have roles in UC.

5-ASA drugs often comprise the initial therapy used to maintain remission in childhood UC. When disease is not well-controlled with ASA drugs, then immunosuppressives would be indicated. Thiopurines (azathioprine or 6-mercaptopurine) are more often utilised, but methotrexate also has a role. Tacrolimus may also have benefits as a maintenance drug to keep control.

10.2 Corticosteroids

CS can be utilised in various routes for active UC. Oral CS in mild to moderate UC may lead to more rapid improvements than those seen in CD. CS (including topical delivery) may have roles in maintenance of remission.

Standard CS therapy to induce remission involves oral prednisone or prednisolone with once daily dosing in the morning (doses as per **Table 2**). Budesonide, which has advantages over prednisone with less systemic absorption and side-effects, has been demonstrated to have a role in the management of ileal CD. The role of budesonide in the management of UC has been considered in several studies. Three of these studies were reviewed together in a recent Cochrane review: budesonide was shown to not be helpful for UC (Sherlock et al 2011). Interestingly, however, budesonide as a MMX preparation was shown to be helpful in a study reported in abstract form at Digestive Diseases Week 2011 (Sandborn et al 2011).

IV Steroids	2 mg/kg/day (max 40 mg/day) once daily in morning (starting dose, then wean as appropriate)
Budesonide	6-9 mg/day (then wean as appropriate)
IV Steroids	Hydrocortisone 2-4 mg/kg/day (q6h); Methylprednisolone 1-1.5 mg/kg/day (q12h)
Sulphasalazine	50-60 mg/kg/day (up to 3-4 grams daily)
5-ASA	30-50 mg/kg/day
Azathioprine	Start 1 - 1.5 mg/kg/day, Increase to approx 2.5 mg/kg/day (max 200 mg/day)
6-MP	Start 1 mg/kg/day, increase to around 1.5 mg/kg/day
Methotrexate	15 mg / m2 (max 25 mg) weekly subcutaneous injection
Tacrolimus	Commence at 0.1 mg/kg/day in 2 divided doses orally
	Usual dose 0.2 mg/kg/day in 2 divided doses (ongoing dose dependant on levels)
Cyclosporin	3-8 mg/kg/dose Q12H

Table 2. Standard doses for drugs used in Paediatric UC

Severe UC often requires the administration of IV CS. Typically this would be given as methyprednisolone, with one or two doses daily, or six-hourly hydrocortisone. Methylprednisolone has the advantage of less mineralocorticoid effects.

One study from Japan has evaluated pulse steroid therapy in children with UC (Kudo et al 2011). This group retrospectively compared outcomes from children with UC treated with conventional methylprednisolone dosing to another group treated with megadose pulse therapy (20-30 mg/kg/day, to max of 1000 mg). Pulse therapy lead to more rapid response, with quicker reduction in PUCDAI scores, without any increase in side-effect profile. Pulse therapy, however, did not alter outcomes over the first 12 months after diagnosis compared to standard therapy. This retrospective data in a small group of patients would require replication and confirmation before broader use of this approach. Other data looking at larger doses of corticosteroids have not suggested benefits.

Topical CS is more often helpful in distal UC, where it has advantages of less systemic absorption and being directed straight to the area of inflammation. Steroid suppositories may be helpful in very distal disease, whereas enemas or foam preparations may have effects in left-sided disease. In these instances, topical CS may have benefits in treating active disease and in maintaining control. However, children may not tolerate the per-rectal administration route.

10.3 Amino-salicylates

This group of therapies includes sulphasalazine and the 5-aminosalicylate (5-ASA) drugs. Delivery routes include oral and rectal (suppository or enema). Packaging of the 5-ASA drugs can provide distribution of the drug at different locations in the gastrointestinal tract. More recent variations of the 5-ASA drugs enable once daily dosing with equivalent efficacy to multiple dosing regimens.

These drugs have roles in the induction and maintenance of remission in UC (Ford et al 2011). Although there are many studies demonstrating efficacy of 5-ASA agents in adults with UC, there are few in children or adolescents. One study demonstrated 80% clinical remission with sulphasalazine at 1, 2 and 3 months and lower response to olsalazine at the same time points (Ferry et al. 1993).

10.4 Thiopurines

Azathioprine or 6-mercaptopurine are the most commonly used immunosuppressives in paediatric IBD. Although well-established as agents that modify disease course in children with moderate-severe CD when used early, there has been little data in paediatric UC. Seventy-five percent of a group of 32 children with UC in a British series received azathioprine (Howarth et al 2007). Recently a prospective multi-centre study evaluated the outcomes of thiopurines in paediatric UC (Hyams et al 2011). This report included 394 children with UC recruited at diagnosis from paediatric centres in USA. One hundred and ninety seven of this group received thiopurines (half within the first 3 months of diagnosis). Due to difficulties in follow-up or other reasons, just 133 of this cohort were re-evaluated after 12 months. Sixty-five of these 133 children were in remission at this time, without CS or rescue therapy.

10.5 Methotrexate

Methotrexate is also well established a second or third line agent for the maintenance of remission in CD. Only recently, however, has it also been considered for the maintenance of remission in UC. Two clinical trials are assessing the role of methotrexate in adult UC (Carbonnel 2011). A recent retrospective report described the outcomes of methotrexate in a group of Canadian children with UC (Willot et al 2011). Four of the 16 children with UC or IBDU were in remission after six months of methotrexate therapy. A further report from Italy evaluated 32 children with UC who were treated with methotrexate (Aloi et al 2010). Response or remission was seen in 72% of the children by 3 months, with 50% at 12 months. Almost all of the children receiving steroids at the start of therapy were able to cease steroids by six months. Both these studies, however, were retrospective assessments of this drug in relatively small cohorts. Prospective studies are required to clarify the role of methotrexate in paediatric UC.

Methotrexate is given as a once weekly subcutaneous injection. Six weeks is usually expected before onset of action, and sixteen weeks would be required before expecting the benefits of the drug. Folate supplementation (but not on the day of methotrexate administration) is required to prevent folate deficiency - this also may decrease upper gut side-effects.

10.6 Infliximab and adalimumab

The anti-Tumour necrosis factor-(TNF) alpha inhibitor Infliximab has been evaluated in adult and paediatric UC.

A recent report demonstrated the benefits of infliximab in paediatric UC (Hyams et al 2010). The outcomes of 52 children recruited prospectively across several sites in USA were followed for a median of 30 months. CS-free remission was seen in 38% of these children at 12 months, with remission in 21% after 24 months. After 2 years of followup, 39% of this group had undergone colectomy. An Italian study has also reviewed their experience with infliximab in children with UC (Cucchiara et al 2008). These 22 children had been treated with infliximab using a three dose induction course and ongoing maintenance dosing (eight weekly). Some of the children had acute severe colitis with no response to CS, whilst others had a protracted course with/without CS dependency. Overall, 12 of the 22 children had full response with CS-free remission after 12 months and 6 others had partial response. Seven children required colectomy (only one during the acute period).

A report in adults with UC unresponsive to CS demonstrated that adalimumab is also safe and effective in this context (Reinisch et al 2011). However, there is not yet data looking at adalimumab or other biologics in paediatric UC.

10.7 Tacrolimus and cyclosporin (CSA)

These calcineurin inhibitors are most typically used as rescue therapy in acute severe UC. Although CSA is favoured in adult protocols, tacrolimus has advantages of oral administration, quicker onset of action and a more tolerable side-effect profile. In the context of acute severe UC, tacrolimus can be used a bridge to allow the introduction of long-term immunosuppressive therapy (such as azathioprine). In addition, tacrolimus may have a role in the management of grumbling colitic symptoms and/or as a longer-term drug to maintain remission.

Tacrolimus was evaluated in an open label multi-centre study as rescue therapy in children with UC (Bousvaros et al 2000). Two thirds of the 14 children responded, but less than half had long-term remission. More recently, a cohort of 46 children managed with tacrolimus was reviewed retrospectively (Watson et al 2011). Ninety-three percent of this group were discharged without requiring colectomy, and the probability of colectomy after tacrolimus therapy was 40% at 26 months. Side-effects in this cohort included hypertension, headaches, seizures, tremor and nephrotoxicity. Although not reported in this cohort, hypomagnesaemia is a further common side-effect. Tacrolimus therapy requires close monitoring of serum levels (aim to achieve 8-10 initially), with ongoing close monitoring of renal function, electrolytes, blood pressure, blood sugar and urinalysis. Magnesium supplementation may be required.

10.8 Exclusive enteral nutrition

This therapy involves the exclusive administration of a liquid diet for 6-8 weeks as sole therapy to induce remission. This therapy is well established as standard induction therapy for newly diagnosed CD in children. Although this therapy has benefits in colonic CD, there is less evidence for a role in UC.

10.9 Novel therapies for UC

Along with the roles of standard medical and surgical therapies has been increasing interest in novel therapies. Foremost of these is probiotic therapies. There is convincing animal and human evidence indicating that modifications to the intestinal flora can prevent or modulate gut inflammation. Recent studies have focused on VSL#3, a high-potency probiotic mixture, in adult and paediatric UC. A recent Italian study in adults with UC demonstrated that

VSL#3 supplementation was safe and effective, with reduction in disease activity scores and symptoms (Tursi et al 2010). An earlier paediatric study evaluated the same probiotic therapy in 29 children with newly-diagnosed active UC using a randomised placebo-controlled design (Miele et al, 2009). Remission was observed in 93% of the children treated with VSL#3, compared to 36% of those who did not receive the probiotic. Less children receiving the probiotic relapsed over the followup period, and no adverse effects were attributed to the probiotic. It is not clear if these findings are specific to VSL#3, or able to be achieved with other probiotics, but are clearly encouraging as a safe and effective therapy for UC.

11. Severe acute colitis

Several recent publications have highlighted key aspects of acute severe colitis in children. Most important of these was a prospective multi-centre study conducted in North America (Turner et al 2010a). This study included 128 children admitted to one of 10 centres for severe UC - both as initial presentation and as subsequent relapse of disease. These children were assessed serially in terms of clinical and laboratory findings, disease activity scores and outcomes, both during hospitalisation and for up to 12 months subsequently. All children were treated with intravenous corticosteroids as initial therapy. Thirty-seven children did not respond to corticosteroids: these children proceeded to receive secondary medical therapy (cyclosporin or infliximab) or underwent colectomy. Overall 9% of children had colectomy by discharge and 19% required this by 12 months follow-up. PUCAI scores calculated during hospitalisation in all children were predictive of response and outcomes. A score of greater than 45 on day 3 of admission predicted lack of response to corticosteroids. In contrast a score of greater than 70 on day 5 guided the start of rescue therapy.

Serial stool samples in this cohort of children were analysed for a suite of faecal inflammatory markers (Turner et al 2010b). All four of the markers (calprotectin, S100A12, M2PK and lactoferrin) were greatly elevated in these children. M2PK provided the best predictive value for response to corticosteroids. However, none of these markers performed better than the PUCAI in this context. A further assessment of a subset of samples from this group of children evaluated faecal osteoprotegrin (OPG): when measured at day three faecal OPG was a good predictor of response to corticosteroids (Sylvester 2011). This marker has previously been evaluated in children with CD (Nahidi et al 2010).

More recently a consensus statement from key European groups has been prepared (Turner et al 2011). This document outlines key recommendations and management pointers for acute severe colitis in children (**Table 3**).

1. Stool evaluation should include standard culture and specific screening for *C difficile*
2. CMV infection should be excluded endoscopically in children with steroid resistant disease
3. Disease activity should be monitored regularly during admission, with frequent assessment of vital signs, completion of PUCAI scores daily and monitoring of key blood tests (ESR, full blood count, albumin and electrolytes) at admission and at subsequent intervals

4. Initial treatment should be with intravenous corticosteroids, with methylprednisolone (1-1.5 mg/kg/day, to max of 60 mgs as 1 or 2 daily doses) favoured due to less mineralocorticoid effect.
5. Antibiotics are not indicated routinely but should be considered when sepsis suspected or when toxic megacolon present
6. There is no evidence for the routine use of prophylactic heparin to prevent thromboembolic events
7. 5-ASA therapies should be interrupted at admission in known patients, or introduction delayed in newly diagnosed patients
8. Regular diet should be continued, but nutritional support (enteral or parenteral) considered if inadequate oral intake. Oral intake should be ceased when surgery imminent and is contraindicated in toxic megacolon.
9. Complications (such as perforation or toxic megacolon) should be considered in children with increasing or severe pain. Narcotics or non-steroidal anti-inflammatory drugs are not recommended in the setting of acute severe colitis.
10. PUCAI scores can be used to monitor response and the need for secondary therapy. A score of >45 at day 3 indicates likely poor response to corticosteroids and a need to prepare for rescue therapy. A score of >65 on day 5 indicates a need to commence rescue therapy on that day. In children with PUCAI scores of between 35 and 60 at day 5, steroids can be continued for a further 2-5 days before secondary therapy should be considered. Children with scores of less than 35 points on day 5 are not likely to require rescue therapy
11. Plain radiographs of the abdomen should be obtained in any child with clinical signs of toxicity and subsequently as indicated. The diagnostic criteria for toxic megacolon comprise radiological evidence colonic dilatation (>=56 mm) along with signs of toxicity. Urgent surgical review is required in all children with toxic megacolon. Conservative management is appropriate if the child has stable vital signs and there are no signs of sepsis. If signs of toxicity worsen, then immediate colectomy should be undertaken. Rescue medical therapies are not indicated in the setting of toxic megacolon.
12. Rescue therapies include medical (infliximab or calcineurin inhibitors) and surgical (colectomy) options.
13. Sequential medical rescue therapies are not recommended in children
14. If colectomy is required in acute severe colitis in children, subtotal colectomy and ilesotomy is recommended. Pouch formation can subsequently be considered.
15. Surgical complications can be reduced by avoiding delays in colectomy to enhance nutrition or to wean corticosteroids and the use of perioperative broad spectrum antibiotic coverage.

Table 3. Recommendations from Consensus statement for the management of acute severe colitis in children (abridged from reference: Turner 2011)

12. Surgical management

Colectomy may be required during childhood in children with UC. Indications include fulminant UC unresponsive to medical therapy, severe colitis complicated by toxic megacolon and/or perforation, chronic colitis unresponsive to medical agents and when pre-cancerous changes develop. One retrospective study has assessed clinical factors that might help in prognosticating the risk of colectomy (Moore et al 2011). In a cohort of 135 children with UC, these authors showed that white blood count and haematocrit values at diagnosis were associated with colectomy at 3 years. A UC Risk Score was derived from these measurements. Risk assessment such as this required further prospective assessment in large numbers of children.

Colectomy may be followed by ileal pouch formation as one or more steps. A two-step procedure might include colectomy and end-ileostomy initially followed by pouch formation. A new pouch may be protected by a defunctioning ileostomy, which is subsequently reversed (third step). Pelvic dissection in young individuals, as required for total colectomy, may be complicated by disruption to pelvic nerves and consequent effects upon fertility.

A condition known as pouchitis may complicate an ileal pouch. Probiotics can be used to prevent or treat pouchitis. Antibiotics (e.g. metronidazole) are also useful for pouchitis.

The outcomes of surgical management of UC in children have been considered in some recent reports. Newby et al reported that 17.6% of 72 children with UC underwent 1 or more major operations over the period of study, with a mean time of 1.92 years to the first procedure (Newby et al 2008). Fraser et al (Fraser et al 2010) retrospectively compared the outcomes of laparoscopic and open colectomy in a group of 44 children aged up 18 years of age. Twenty-seven of this group were diagnosed with UC - the remainder had various other surgical diagnoses. There were no differences between the technique in terms of postoperative abscess or sepsis, would infection of small bowel obstruction. The children having laparoscopic ileoanal reanastomosis and pouch formation had less pouchitis than those having open pouch formation (p=0.03).

A second study (Lillehei et al 2010) evaluated QOL scores in children undergoing proctocolectomy and pouch formation. The children with UC and their parents reported low QOL scores pre-operatively that improved substantially with resection. This report did not evaluate other aspects of the outcomes of surgical intervention.

13. Transition of adolescents with UC to adult services

One of the last components of the management of adolescents with UC is preparing them for the move on from paediatric care to adult care. This transition is increasingly recognised as an important step in the overall management of young people with chronic diseases, such as UC (Viner 2008). The move from a family-focused multi-disciplinary model of care in the paediatric setting to the adult setting that typically features an individual-focused approach that may be office based and more rigid, with expectations of patient involvement. Preparation for this transition can include review of understanding of medications, knowledge of key aspects of disease management, and practical aspects of health care (such as renewal of scripts, learning how to organise appointments and health benefit applications if appropriate). A successful transition should lead to a more confident young person able to better care for their own health and willing to take charge of their care. Further, it should also mean that less young people "fall between the cracks", and ultimately lead to better quality of life and health outcomes.

14. Conclusions

Children and adolescents should be considered a distinct and special group of patients with numerous important clinical features, and with particular management needs and requirements. At this point in time, genetic evaluation is not part of routine clinical management. In time, however, analysis of mutations in key relevant genes will likely be considered routine. Such developments will serve to further differentiate paediatric UC from the condition in older individuals and perhaps will also assist in defining clinical subgroups that may indicate specialised therapeutic needs and/or provide key prognostic information.

15. References

Aloi M, Di Nardo G, Conte F, Mazzeo L, Cavallari N, Nuti F, Cucchiara S, Stronati L. (2010) Methotrexate in paediatric ulcerative colitis: a retrospective survey at a single tertiary referral centre. *Aliment Pharmacol Ther.* 32:1017-22.

Anderson CA, Boucher G, Lees CW, Franke A, D'Amato M, Taylor KD, Lee JC, Goyette P, Imielinski M, Latiano A, Lagacé C, Scott R, Amininejad L, Bumpstead S, Baidoo L, Baldassano RN, Barclay M, Bayless TM, Brand S, Büning C, Colombel JF, Denson LA, De Vos M, Dubinsky M, Edwards C, Ellinghaus D, Fehrmann RS, Floyd JA, Florin T, Franchimont D, Franke L, Georges M, Glas J, Glazer NL, Guthery SL, Haritunians T, Hayward NK, Hugot JP, Jobin G, Laukens D, Lawrance I, Lémann M, Levine A, Libioulle C, Louis E, McGovern DP, Milla M, Montgomery GW, Morley KI, Mowat C, Ng A, Newman W, Ophoff RA, Papi L, Palmieri O, Peyrin-Biroulet L, Panés J, Phillips A, Prescott NJ, Proctor DD, Roberts R, Russell R, Rutgeerts P, Sanderson J, Sans M, Schumm P, Seibold F, Sharma Y, Simms LA, Seielstad M, Steinhart AH, Targan SR, van den Berg LH, Vatn M, Verspaget H, Walters T, Wijmenga C, Wilson DC, Westra HJ, Xavier RJ, Zhao ZZ, Ponsioen CY, Andersen V, Torkvist L, Gazouli M, Anagnou NP, Karlsen TH, Kupcinskas L, Sventoraityte J, Mansfield JC, Kugathasan S, Silverberg MS, Halfvarson J, Rotter JI, Mathew CG, Griffiths AM, Gearry R, Ahmad T, Brant SR, Chamaillard M, Satsangi J, Cho JH, Schreiber S, Daly MJ, Barrett JC, Parkes M, Annese V, Hakonarson H, Radford-Smith G, Duerr RH, Vermeire S, Weersma RK, Rioux JD. (2011). Meta-analysis identifies 29 additional ulcerative colitis risk loci, increasing the number of confirmed associations to 47. *Nat Genet.* 43: 246-52.

Bastida G, Beltran B. (2011) Ulcerative colitis in smokers, non-smokers and ex-smokers. *World J Gastro.* 17: 2740-7.

Benchimol EI, Fortinsky KJ, Gozdyra P, Van den Heuvel M, Van Limbergen J, Griffiths AM. (2011). Epidemiology of pediatric inflammatory bowel disease: a systematic review of international trends. *Inflamm Bowel Dis.* 17:423-39.

Benchimol EI, Guttmann A, Griffiths AM, Rabeneck L, Mack DR, Brill H, Howard J, Guan J, To T. (2009) Increasing incidence of paediatric inflammatory bowel disease in Ontario, Canada: evidence from health administrative data. *Gut.* 58: 1490-7.

Berrebi D, Languepin J, Ferkdadji L, Foussat A, De Lagausie P, Paris R, Emilie D, Mougenot JF, Cezard JP, Navarro J, Peuchmaur M. (2003). Cytokines, chemokine receptors, and homing molecule distribution in the rectum and stomach of pediatric patients with ulcerative colitis. *J Pediatr Gastroenterol Nutr.* 37:300-8.

Bousvaros A, Kirschner B, Werlin S, Parker-Hartigan L, Daum F, Freeman K, Balint J, Day AS, Griffiths A, Zurakowski D, Ferry G, Leichtner AM. (2000) Oral tacrolimus treatment of severe colitis in children. *J Pediatr.* 137:794-9.

Broide E, Dotan I, Weiss B, Wilschanski M, Yerushalmi B, Klar A, Levine A. (2011) Idiopathic pancreatitis preceding the diagnosis of inflammatory bowel disease is more frequent in pediatric patients. *J Pediatr Gastroenterol Nutr.* 52:714-7.

Carbonnel F. (2011). Methotrexate: A Drug of the Future in Ulcerative Colitis? *Curr Drug Targets.* Apr 5. [Epub ahead of print]

Cho JH, Brant SR. (2011). Recent insights into the genetics of inflammatory bowel disease. *Gastroenterology. 140: 1704-12.*

Colombel JF, Rutgeerts P. Reinisch W, Esser D, Wang Y, Lang Y, Marano CW, Strauss R, Oddens BJ, Feagen BG, Hanauer SB, Lichtenstein GR, Present D, Sands BE, Sandborn WJ. (2011). Early mucosal healing with infliximab is associated with improved long-term clinical outcomes in ulcerative colitis. *Gastroenterology,* June 29. [Epub ahead of print].

Costa F, Mumolo MG, Ceccarelli L, Bellini M, Romano MR, Sterpi C, Ricchiuti A, Marchi S, Bottai M. (2005). Calprotectin is a stronger predictive marker of relapse in ulcerative colitis than in Crohn's disease. *Gut.* 54:364-8.

Cucchiara S, Romeo E, Viola F, Cottone M, Fontana M, Lombardi G, Rutigliano V, de'Angelis GL, Federici T. (2008). Infliximab for pediatric ulcerative colitis: a retrospective Italian multicenter study. *Dig Liver Dis.* 40 Suppl 2:S260-4.

Dotson JL, Hyams JS, Markowitz J, LeLeiko NS, Mack DR, Evans JS, Pfefferkorn MD, Griffiths AM, Otley AR, Bousvaros A, Kugathasan S, Rosh JR, Keljo D, Carvalho RS, Tomer G, Mamula P, Kay MH, Kerzner B, Oliva-Hemker M, Langton CR, Crandall W. (2010). Extraintestinal manifestations of pediatric inflammatory bowel disease and their relation to disease type and severity. *J Pediatr Gastroenterol Nutr.* 51:140-5.

Ferry GD, Kirschner BS, Grand RJ, et al. (1993). Olsalazine versus sulfasalazine in mild to moderate childhood ulcerative colitis: results of the Pediatric Gastroenterology Collaborative Research Group Clinical Trial. *J Pediatr Gastroenterol Nutr.* 17:32–8.

Ford AC, Achkar JP, Khan KJ, Kane SV, Talley NJ, Marshall JK, Moayyedi P. (2011). Efficacy of 5-aminosalicylates in ulcerative colitis: a systematic review and meta-analysis. *Am J Gastroenterol.* 106: 601-16.

Fraser JD, Garey CL, Laituri CA, Sharp RJ, Ostlei DJ, St Peter SD. (2010). Oucomes of laparoscopic and open total colectomy in the paediatric population. *J Laparoendosc Adv Surg Tech A.* 20: 659-60.

Gearry RB, Richardson AK, Frampton CM, Dodgshun AJ, Barclay ML. (2010). Population-based cases control study of inflammatory bowel disease risk factors. *J Gastroenterol Hepatol.* 25:325-33.

Goh KL, Xiao S-D. (2009). Inflammatory bowel disease: a survey of the epidemiology in Asia. *J Dig Dis.* 10: 1-6

Gower-Rousseau C, Dauchet L, Vernier-Massouille G, Tilloy E, Brazier F, Merle V, Dupas JL, Savoye G, Balde M, Marti R, Lerebours E, Cortot A, Salomez JL, Turck D, Colombel JF. (2009). The natural history of pediatric ulcerative colitis: a population-based cohort study. *Am J Gastroenterol.* 104: 2080-8.

Griffiths AM, Hugot J-P. (2004). Crohn Disease. Chapter 41, Pediatric Gastrointestinal Disease, 4th Edition. Eds: Walker A, Goulet O, Kleinman RE, et al., BC Decker, Hamilton Ontario.

Henderson P, Hansen R, Cameron FL, Gerasimidis K, Rogers P, Bisset WM, Reynish EL, Drummond HE, Anderson NH, Van Limbergen J, Russell RK, Satsangi J, Wilson DC. (2011b). Rising incidence of pediatric inflammatory bowel disease in Scotland. *Inflamm Bowel Dis.* Jun 17. doi: 10.1002

Henderson P, van Limbergen JE, Wilson DC, Satsangi J, Russell RK. (2011a). Genetics of childhood-onset Inflammatory Bowel Disease. *Inflamm Bowel Dis.* 17: 346-361

Hori K, Ikeuchi H, Nakano H, Uchino M, Tomita T, Ohda Y, Hida N, Matsumoto T, Fukuda Y, Miwa H. (2008). Gastroduodenitis associated with ulcerative colitis. *J Gastroenterol.* 43:193-201.

Howarth LJ, Wiskin AE, Griffiths DM, Afzal NA, Beattie RM. (2007). Outcome of childhood ulcerative colitis at 2 years. *Acta Paediatr.* 96: 1790-3

Hyams J, Markowitz J, Lerer T, Griffiths A, Mack D, Bousvaros A, Otley A, Evans J, Pfefferkorn M, Rosh J, Rothbaum R, Kugathasan S, Mezoff A, Wyllie R, Tolia V, delRosario JF, Moyer MS, Oliva-Hemker M, Leleiko N. (2006). Pediatric Inflammatory Bowel Disease Collaborative Research Group. The natural history of corticosteroid therapy for ulcerative colitis in children. *Clin Gastroenterol Hepatol.* 4:1118-23.

Hyams JS, Lerer T, Griffiths A, Pfefferkorn M, Stephens M, Evans J, Otley A, Carvalho R, Mack D, Bousvaros A, Rosh J, Grossman A, Tomer G, Kay M, Crandall W, Oliva-Hemker M, Keljo D, LeLeiko N, Markowitz J; Pediatric Inflammatory Bowel Disease Collaborative Research Group. (2010). Outcome following infliximab therapy in children with ulcerative colitis. *Am J Gastroenterol.* 105:1430-6.

Hyams JS, Lerer T, Mack D, Bousvaros A, Griffiths A, Rosh J, Otley A, Evans J, Stephens M, Kay M, Keljo D, Pfefferkorn M, Saeed S, Crandall W, Michail S, Kappelman MD, Grossman A, Samson C, Sudel B, Oliva-Hemker M, Leleiko N, Markowitz J. (2011). Pediatric Inflammatory Bowel Disease Collaborative Research Group Registry. Outcome following thiopurine use in children with ulcerative colitis: a prospective multicenter registry study. *Am J Gastroenterol.* 106:981-7.

IBD Working Group of the European Society for Paediatric Gastroenterology, Hepatology and Nutrition. (2005). Inflammatory bowel disease in children and adolescents: Recommendations for diagnosis – The Porto criteria. *J Pediatr Gastroenterol Nutr.* 41: 1-7.

Ishige T, Tomomasa T, Takebayashi T, Asakura K, Watanabe M, Suzuki T, Miyazawa R, Arakawa H. (2010). Inflammatory bowel disease in children: epidemiological analysis of the nationwide IBD registry in Japan. *J Gastroenterol.* 45: 911-7.

Kudo T, Nagata S, Ohtani K, Fujii T, Wada M, Haruna H, Shoji H, Ohtsuka Y, Shimizu T, Yamashiro Y. (2011). Pulse steroids as induction therapy for children with ulcerative colitis. *Pediatr Int.* (Epub ahead of print)

Kugathasan S, Dubinsky MC, Keljo D, Moyer MS, Rufo PA, Wyllie R, Zachos M, Hyams J. (2005). Severe colitis in children. *J Pediatr Gastroenterol Nutr.* 41:375-85.

Kugathasan S, Judd RH, Hoffmann RG, Heikenen J, Telega G, Khan F, Weisdorf-Schindele S, San Pablo W, Perrault J, Park R, Yaffe M, Brown C, Rivera-Bennett MT, Halabi I, Martinez A, Blank E, Werlin SL, Rudolph CD, Binion DG. (2003). Epidemiologic and clinical characteristics of children with newly diagnosed inflammatory bowel disease in Wisconsin: a statewide population-based study. *J Pediatr.* 143: 525-31.

Lehtinen P, Ashorn M, Iltanen S, Jauhola R, Jauhonen P, Kolho K-L, Auvinen A. (2011). Incidence Trends of Pediatric Inflammatory Bowel Disease in Finland, 1987–2003, a Nationwide Study. *Inflamm Bowel Dis.* 17:1778–1783)

Levine A, Griffiths A, Markowitz J, Wilson DC, Turner D, Russell RK, Fell J, Ruemmele FM, Walters T, Sherlock M, Dubinsky M, Hyams JS. (2011). Pediatric modification of the Montreal classification for inflammatory bowel disease: the Paris classification. *Inflamm Bowel Dis.* 7:1314-21.

Lillehei CW, Masek BJ, Shamberger RC. (2010). Prospective study of health-related quality of life and restorative proctocolectomy in children. *Dis Colon Rectum.* 53: 1388-92.

Long MD, Crandall WV, Leibowitz IH, Duffy L, Del Rosario F, Kim SC, Integlia MJ, Berman J, Grunow J, Colletti RB, Schoen BT, Patel AS, Baron H, Israel E, Russell G, Ali S, Herfarth HH, Martin C, Kappelman MD. (2010). Prevalence and Epidemiology of Overweight and Obesity in Children with Inflammatory Bowel Disease. *Inflamm Bowel Dis.* In press

Mack DR, Langton C, Markowitz J et al. (2007). Laboratory values for children with newly diagnosed inflammatory bowel disease. *Pediatrics.* 119: 1113-9.

Mahid SS, Minor KS, Stromberg AJ, Galandiuk S. (2007). Active and passive smoking in childhood is related to the development of inflammatory bowel disease. *Inflamm Bowel Dis.* 13: 431-8

Man SM, Zhang L, Day AS, Leach ST, Lemberg DA, Mitchell H. (2010). Campylobacter concisus and other Campylobacter species in children with newly diagnosed Crohn's disease. *Inflamm Bowel Dis.* 16:1008-16.

Martin De Carpi J, Vila V, Varea V. (2011). Application of the Porto criteria for the diagnosis of paediatric inflammatory bowel disease in a paediatric reference centre. *An Pediatr (Barc).* E pub before print.

Miele E, Pascarella F, Giannetti E, Quaglietta L, Baldassano RN, Staiano A. (2009). Effect of a probiotic preparation (VSL#3) on induction and maintenance of remission in children with ulcerative colitis. *Am J Gastroenterol.* 104:437-43.

Mukhopadhya I, Thomson JM, Hansen R, Berry SH, El-Omar EM, Hold GL. (2011). Detection of Campylobacter concisus and other Campylobacter species in colonic biopsies from adults with ulcerative colitis. *PLoS One.* 6: e21490.

Nahidi L, Leach ST, Sidler MA, Levin A, Lemberg DA, Day AS. (2011). Osteoprotegerin expression in paediatric Crohn's disease and modification by exclusive enteral nutrition. *Inflamm Bowel Dis,* 17: 516-523.

Newby EA, Croft NM, Green M, Hassan K, Heuschkel RB, Jenkins H, Casson DH. (2008). Natural history of paediatric inflammatory bowel diseases over a 5-year follow-up:

a retrospective review of data from the register of paediatric inflammatory bowel diseases. *J Pediatr Gastroenterol Nutr*. 46:539-45.

North American Society of Pediatric Gastroenterology, Hepatology and Nutrition; Colitis Foundation of America, Bousvaros A, Antonioli DA, Coletti RB, Dubinsky MC, Glickman JN, Gold BD, Griffiths AM, Jevon GP, Higuchi LM, Hyams JS, Kirschner BS, Kugasthasan S, Baldassano RN, Russo PA. (2007). Differentiating ulcerative colitis from Crohn disease in children and young adults: report of a working group of the North American Society for Pediatric Gastroenterology, Hepatology and Nutrition and the Crohn's and Colitis Foundation of America. *J Pediatr Gastroenterol Nutr*.44: 653-74.

Rajwal SR, Puntis JW, McClean P et al. (2004). Endoscopic rectal sparing in children with untreated ulcerative colitis. *J Pediatr Gastroenterol Nutr*. 38: 66-9.

Ramasundara M, Leach ST, Lemberg DA, Day AS. (2009). Defensins and Inflammation: the role of defensins in Inflammatory Bowel Disease. *J Gastroenterol Hepatol*, 24:202-8.

Reinisch W, Sandborn WJ, Hommes DW, D'Haens G, Hanauer S, Schreiber S, Panaccione R, Fedorak RN, Tighe MB, Huang B, Kampman W, Lazar A, Thakkar R. (2011). Adalimumab for induction of clinical remission in moderately to severely active ulcerative colitis: results of a randomised controlled trial. *Gut*. 60:780-7.

Sandborn WJ, Travis S, Danese S, Kupcinskas, Alexeeva O, Moro L, Ballard D, Bleker WF, Kriesel D, Yeung P. (2011). Budesonide-MMx 9 mg for induction of remission of mild-moderate ulcerative colitis: data from a multicentrer, randomised, double-blind, placebo-controlled study in Europe, Russia, Israel and Australia. *Digestive Diseases Week*, Abstract 292.

Sawczenko A, Sandhu BK. (2003). Presenting features of inflammatory bowel disease in Great Britain and Ireland. *Arch Dis Child*. 88:995-1000.

Sherlock ME, Seow CH, Steinhart AH, Griffiths AM. (2010). Oral budesonide for induction of remission in ulcerative colitis. *Cochrane Database Syst Rev*. 6;:CD007698.

Silverberg MS, Satsangi J, Ahmad T, Arnott ID, Bernstein CN, Brant SR, Caprilli R, Colombel JF, Gasche C, Geboes K, Jewell DP, Karban A, Loftus Jr EV, Peña AS, Riddell RH, Sachar DB, Schreiber S, Steinhart AH, Targan SR, Vermeire S, Warren BF. (2005). Toward an integrated clinical, molecular and serological classification of inflammatory bowel disease: Report of a Working Party of the 2005 Montreal World Congress of Gastroenterology. *Can J Gastroenterol*. 19 Suppl A:5-36.

Sondike SB, McGuire E, Kugathasan S. (2004). Weight status in pediatric IBD patients at the time of diagnosis: effects of the obesity epidemic. *J Pediatr Gastroenterol Nutr*. 39 Suppl 1: S317.

Sylvester FA, Turner D, Draghi A 2nd, Uuosoe K, McLernon R, Koproske K, Mack DR, Crandall WV, Hyams JS, Leleiko NS, Griffiths AM. (2011). Fecal osteoprotegerin may guide the introduction of second-line therapy in hospitalized children with ulcerative colitis. *Inflamm Bowel Dis*. 17:1726-30

Thompson AI, Lees CW. (2011). Genetics of Ulcerative Colitis. *Inflamm Bowel Dis*. 17:831–848

Tsampalieros A, Griffiths AM, Barrowman N, Mack DR. (2011). Use of C-Reactive Protein in Children with Newly Diagnosed Inflammatory bowel disease. *J Pediatrics*, [Epub ahead of print].

Turner D, Hyams J, Markowitz J, Lerer T, Mack DR, Evans J, Pfefferkorn M, Rosh J, Kay M, Crandall W, Keljo D, Otley AR, Kugathasan S, Carvalho R, Oliva-Hemker M, Langton C, Mamula P, Bousvaros A, LeLeiko N, Griffiths AM. (2009). Pediatric IBD Collaborative Research Group. Appraisal of the Pediatric Ulcerative colitis activity index (PUCAI). *Inflamm Bowel Dis.* 15:1218-23.

Turner D, Leach ST, Mack D, Uusoue K, Hyams J , Leleiko N, Walters TD, Crandall W, Markowitz J, Otley AR, Griffiths AM, Day AS. (2010b). Fecal calprotectin, lactoferrin, M2-pyruvate kinase, and S100A12 in severe acute ulcerative colitis: a prospective multicentre comparison of predicting outcomes and monitoring response. *Gut.* 59: 1207-12

Turner D, Mack D, Leleiko N, Walters TD, Uusoue K, Leach ST, Day AS, Crandall W, Silverberg MS, Markowitz J, Otley AR, Keljo D, Mamula P, Kugathasan S, Hyams J, Griffiths AM. (2010a). Severe pediatric ulcerative colitis: a prospective multicenter study of outcomes and predictors of response. *Gastroenterology.* 138:2282-91

Turner D, Otley AR, Mack D, Hyams J, de Bruijne J, Uusoue K, Walters TD, Zachos M, Mamula P, Beaton DE, Steinhart AH, Griffiths AM. (2007). Development, validation, and evaluation of a pediatric ulcerative colitis activity index: a prospective multicenter study. *Gastroenterology.* 133:423-32

Turner D, Travis SP, Griffiths AM, Ruemmele FM, Levine A, Benchimol EI, Dubinsky M, Alex G, Baldassano RN, Langer JC, Shamberger R, Hyams JS, Cucchiara S, Bousvaros A, Escher JC, Markowitz J, Wilson DC, van Assche G, Russell RK. (2011). European Crohn's and Colitis Organization; Porto IBD Working Group, European Society of Pediatric Gastroenterology, Hepatology, and Nutrition. Consensus for managing acute severe ulcerative colitis in children: a systematic review and joint statement from ECCO, ESPGHAN, and the Porto IBD Working Group of ESPGHAN. *Am J Gastroenterol.* 106:574-88.

Turner D, Walsh CM, Benchimol EI, Mann EH, Thomas KE, Chow C, McLernon RA, Walters TD, Swales J, Steinhart AH, Griffiths AM. (2008). Severe paediatric ulcerative colitis: incidence, outcomes and optimal timing for second-line therapy. *Gut.* 57:331-8.

Tursi A, Brandimarte G, Papa A, Giglio A, Elisei W, Giorgetti GM, Forti G, Morini S, Hassan C, Pistoia MA, Modeo ME, Rodino' S, D'Amico T, Sebkova L, Sacca' N, Di Giulio E, Luzza F, Imeneo M, Larussa T, Di Rosa S, Annese V, Danese S, Gasbarrini A. (2010). Treatment of relapsing mild-to-moderate ulcerative colitis with the probiotic VSL#3 as adjunctive to a standard pharmaceutical treatment: a double-blind, randomized, placebo-controlled study. *Am J Gastroenterol.* 105:2218-27.

Van der Heide F, Wassenaar M, van der Linde K, Spoelstra P, Klebeuker JH, Dijkstra G. (2011). Effects of active and passive smoking on Crohn's disease and ulcerative colitis in a cohort from a regional hospital. *Eur J Gastroenterol Hepatol.* 23: 255-61

Van Limbergen J, Russell RK, Drummond HE, Aldhous MC, Round NK, Nimmo ER, Smith L, Gillett PM, McGrogan P, Weaver LT, Bisset WM, Mahdi G, Arnott ID, Satsangi J, Wilson DC. (2008). Definition of phenotypic characteristics of childhood-onset inflammatory bowel disease. *Gastroenterology.* 135: 1114-22.

Viner RM. (2008).Transition of care from paediatric to adult services: one part of improved health services for adolescents. *Arch Dis Child.* 93: 160-3.

Watson S, Pensabene L, Mitchell P, Bousvaros A. (2011). Outcomes and adverse events in children and young adults undergoing tacrolimus therapy for steroid-refractory colitis. *Inflamm Bowel Dis.*17:22-9.

Willot S, Noble A, Deslandres C. (2011). Methotrexate in the treatment of inflammatory bowel disease: An 8-year retrospective study in a Canadian pediatric IBD center. *Inflamm Bowel Dis.* Feb 18. doi: 10.1002/ibd.21653. [Epub ahead of print]

Part 3

From Bench to Bedside

10

Animal Models of Colitis: Lessons Learned, and Their Relevance to the Clinic

Matthew Barnett[1] and Alan Fraser[2]
[1]*Food Nutrition & Health Team, Food & Bio-based Products, AgResearch Limited, Grasslands Research Centre, Palmerston North,*
[2]*Department of Medicine, Faculty of Medical and Health Sciences, The University of Auckland, Private Bag 92019, Auckland,*
[1,2]*Nutrigenomics New Zealand (NuNZ) collaboration between The University of Auckland, AgResearch Limited, and Plant & Food Research*
New Zealand

1. Introduction

The term 'Inflammatory Bowel Disease' (IBD) refers to conditions characterized by chronic inflammation of the gastrointestinal tract, including ulcerative colitis (UC) and Crohn's disease (CD). UC and CD have distinct pathologic features, for example the location, depth and severity of inflammation. For UC, inflammation is confined to the colon and rectum, is continuous, and is superficial, affecting only the mucosal layer of the intestinal wall. In contrast, the inflammation seen in CD can affect any part of the gastrointestinal tract from mouth to anus, is typically discontinuous or 'patchy', and involves all layers of the intestinal wall (Abraham and Cho, 2009). In spite of these differences, there is also overlapping pathology, suggesting some common causal factors and potential treatments.

The exact cause of IBD is still unclear, although it appears to involve a complex interaction between genetic susceptibility and environmental triggers including the resident microbial population of the intestinal tract (Abraham and Cho, 2009). The gastrointestinal tract uses a system of tolerance and controlled inflammation to limit the response to dietary or bacterially-derived antigens in the intestinal tract. When this complex system breaks down, either by a chemical or pathogenic insult in a genetically predisposed individual, the resulting innate immune response may lead to IBD. Although the aetiopathogenesis of IBD remains unsolved, current evidence indicates that increased activation of T cells, and an imbalance of Treg and Th1, Th2 and Th17 cells play important roles (Sanchez-Munoz et al., 2008). Activation of macrophages also seems to be important, with increased production of the macrophage-derived cytokines such as TNF-alpha, IL-1 and IL-6 contributing to the observed inflammation. The triggering factor(s) are still to be elucidated, although host response to microbial pathogens includes self-defense mechanisms including defensins, pattern recognition receptors and Toll-like receptors; this suggests there may be an element of "self" recognition triggering the immune response (Strober et al., 2002). Neuroimmunomodulation in IBD is another interesting possible mechanism with its implications relating to the influence of the brain-gut axis on the perpetuation of intestinal inflammation (Tsianos and Katsanos, 2009).

Evidence for a genetic component comes from various sources such as twin studies and familial aggregation, which suggest that CD has a stronger genetic component than UC (Halfvarson et al., 2003). A number of genome-wide association studies (GWAS) have also identified several key gene variants which occur at a higher rate in people with IBD compared with controls who do not have any gastrointestinal symptoms (Barrett et al., 2008). These findings have led to significant recent progress in the understanding of the genetic component of IBD. Relevant genes and pathways have been well characterized for CD, such as innate immunity, adaptive immunity, and more recently autophagy (Massey and Parkes, 2007; Van Limbergen et al., 2009). The part played by autophagy had not been recognized prior to the comprehensive GWAS data, but these data have allowed research to focus on this pathway with a resultant significant increase in understanding of how it may contribute to IBD pathogenesis (Brest et al., 2010). There is also overlap with other diseases, particularly auto-immune diseases, showing genetic variants in the same pathways (Lees et al., 2011).

The genetic component of UC is less well understood than CD, but it seems likely that variants in mucosal barrier function genes (ECM1, CDH1, HNF4α, and laminin B1) are associated with increased risk of UC, and impaired IL10 signalling appears to be a key pathway in intestinal inflammation (Thompson and Lees, 2011). It has been observed that there are currently ninety nine published IBD susceptibility loci (Lees et al., 2011), and genetic variants contributing to both CD and UC have recently been reviewed (Paul et al., 2011).

Recent advances in understanding the genetic contribution to IBD have served to highlight the genetic complexity of the disease, as reflected by the large number of genes potentially implicated in disease pathogenesis or risk. The analysis becomes more complex as risk genes for one ethnic group may not be replicated in another. This has been shown several times, with gene variants identified in populations of European origin showing only limited agreement in, for example, North Indian (Juyal et al., 2011), Indian (Mahurkar et al., 2010), and Japanese (Nakagome et al., 2010) population groups. A combination of the genetic and pathological complexity has contributed to the relatively poor understanding of IBD. The widely varying phenotype suggests many different pathways for the disease, but attempts to sub-classify CD and UC in clinical terms have only been partially successful. This lack of clarity in clinical classification has hampered attempts at genotype-phenotype associations, which has in turn contributed to difficulties in establishing appropriate clinical interventions.

Recent studies have highlighted the relationship between disease and the intestinal microbiota, with the suggestion that an inappropriate immune/inflammatory response to normal intestinal bacteria may be a key triggering factor (Nell et al., 2010). Environment may also play an important role, with diet in particular having an influence, if not in the initiation of the disease, then certainly in the maintenance and/or amelioration of disease symptoms. As part of a long-term research project (Nutrigenomics New Zealand (NuNZ); www.nutrigenomics.org.nz) we have identified a number of foods which are perceived by people with IBD as being either detrimental or beneficial in terms of managing the symptoms of both CD and UC (Petermann et al., 2009b) or show evidence of ameliorating intestinal inflammation in animal studies (Knoch et al., 2009; Nones et al., 2009; Knoch et al., 2010).

There is a very real importance in seeking answers to the effective treatment of IBD because it is such a debilitating condition, and its prevalence is increasing (Cosnes et al., 2011). There is reduced quality of life from continuing disease activity and significant long-term complications that develop with persistent intestinal inflammation. There is clearly an as-yet unmet clinical need due to limitations of current treatments. These tend to rely on the use of non-specific anti-inflammatory agents (such as 5-aminosalicytic acid and corticosteroids) and immunosuppressive drugs that may cause severe side effects, and in a significant percentage of the patients do not provide appreciable benefits (Grimm, 2009). Other approaches such as targeted interruption of the inflammatory cascade using anti-TNF monoclonal antibodies have been very successful, but greater understanding of the inflammatory process is required to identify other pivotal points in the relevant pathways that may be blocked by similar monoclonal antibodies. Surgical removal of diseased portions of the gastro-intestinal tract can be effective but highlights the failure of medical treatment to prevent the long-term consequences of chronic inflammation.

IBD may represent a heterogenic group of diseases that share similar pathologies and mechanisms of tissue damage, but are initiated by different events and characterized by a variety of immune abnormalities (Tsianos and Katsanos, 2009). A variety of mouse models of IBD have been used. This chapter will discuss if this represents the complexity and heterogeneity of IBD or if the multiple models simply reflect the failure of any one model to truly recreate the human disease. Research using these models has attempted to better understand disease pathogenesis and treatment, and to investigate the complex interactions that may be contributing to the pathogenesis. A better understanding of all these factors will provide new insights into the mechanisms by which intestinal inflammation is inappropriately triggered, and provide new targets for medical therapies.

In this chapter, we will review some of the key animal models used in IBD research, consider some of the findings from this research, and finally and most importantly discuss whether these research findings are being applied in a clinical setting to make a real impact for people with IBD.

2. Animal models of IBD

Animal models of IBD have been used for over fifty years. Early models resulted from the observation that a variety of laboratory animals fed extracts from certain species of seaweed displayed similar symptoms to human IBD (Marcus and Watt, 1969). Subsequent refinement and development of this model led to a variety of chemically-induced models. More recently, gene variants relevant to IBD have been incorporated into animal models (primarily mice and rats) and these have been used extensively (Jurjus et al., 2004). These models have recently been comprehensively reviewed in the context of the role of intestinal bacteria in the development of IBD (Nell et al., 2010).

Clinical features in animal models that are of relevance to human IBD include weight loss, anaemia, diarrhoea, visible or occult blood, and sometimes mucus in the faeces. Pathologically there are similarities such as ulceration of variable extent and largely confined to the mucosa, some loss of haustration (i.e., disappearance of the horizontal folds of the colon), granularity of the mucosa along with pseudo-polyps and polypoidal formations (UC features), as well as strictures leading to intestinal obstruction (a feature of CD). Histological features in common are acute, subacute, and chronic inflammatory changes in the mucosa, with occasional crypt abscesses and cystic dilatation or distortion of mucosal glands, mucosal ulceration in various stages of progression and healing, and hyperplastic changes of the glandular epithelium.

Animal models of IBD have significant advantages - one can investigate not only factors concerned in pathogenesis, but also the secondary effects of ulceration, e.g., liver changes, effects on protein metabolism, electrolytic changes in the cellular and extracellular spaces, and other systemic complications. They may also be used to study the influence of drugs or other potential therapies on the pathogenesis and course of the disease process. However, none of the current IBD models in itself constitutes a faithful equivalent for the human diseases (this will be discussed in more detail in the final section of this chapter). It may therefore be essential to evaluate the effect of any candidate therapies in several IBD models. The wide variety of models of IBD includes chemically-induced models, adoptive transfer models, and genetically modified models such as gene knockouts and transgenic animals. We will consider each of these types of model as they apply to IBD, focusing in particular on those models with a genetic basis, describing some of our work using the *Il10*$^{-/-}$and Mdr1a models and, more recently, the *Nod2*^{2939iC} model.

2.1 Chemically induced models of IBD

A variety of agents have been used as inducers of colitis in animal models, including carragenin (Moyana and Lalonde, 1990), acetic acid (MacPherson and Pfeiffer, 1978), and very recently, sodium hydroxide (Kocak et al., 2011). While predominantly used in rodents, compounds such as these have also been used to develop colitis models in dogs (Shibata et al., 1993) and rabbits (Depoortere et al., 2004). The two most widely used chemicals used to induce IBD in such models are 2,4,6-trinitrobenzene sulfonic acid (TNBS) and dextran sodium sulphate (DSS). Both act via acute destruction of the intestinal barrier, although TNBS more closely mimics CD, and DSS UC (Alex et al., 2009). We will consider these two compounds in greater depth as examples of chemically-induced models of colitis.

2.1.1 DSS

DSS, $(C_6H_7Na_3O_{14}S_3)_n$, is a polyanionic derivative of dextran, and is used for such diverse applications as selective precipitation of lipoproteins (Burstein et al., 1970), acceleration of probe hybridization to membrane-immobilized DNA (Wahl et al., 1979), and the release of DNA from DNA-histone complexes (Kent et al., 1958). Its use in animal models is more recent, and it has been widely used in both mice and rats in the context of colorectal cancer (Ishioka et al., 1987) in addition to its role as a model of intestinal colitis (Okayasu et al., 1990) which we are considering here.

DSS is most commonly administered in the drinking water, often as a 3% solution (Johansson et al., 2010), although it can also be administered rectally. This compound results in inflammation in wild-type animals that starts distally after about five days and is confined to the colonic mucosa (Fig.1, [A–C]). How DSS initiates the colonic inflammation is not well understood despite its wide use, although a recent study investigating DSS both *in vitro* (effect on the inner mucus layer secreted by mucosal explants) and *in vivo* (mice given a 3% DSS solution) showed that DSS has a direct effect on the inner mucus layer, allowing bacteria to penetrate this layer before any signs of inflammation could be observed. The authors concluded that a lack of the inner colon mucus layer may be an initial event in the development which allows bacteria to reach the epithelial cells and thus trigger the characteristic inflammatory reaction (Johansson et al., 2010).

As well as being used in wild-type mice, DSS is also used in some genetic models of IBD, which while being genetically predisposed to inflammation still require this challenge in order to trigger an inflammatory response. This is the case for the *Nod2*^{2939iC} mouse model (described in more detail in section 2.3.3) in which DSS treatment led to more severe colonic inflammation and ulceration than wild-type mice (Maeda et al., 2005).

2.1.2 TNBS

TNBS is a nitroaryl oxidizing acid with extreme oxidising properties. TNBS dissolved in ethanol induces severe colonic damage, which is characterized by areas of necrosis surrounded by areas of acute inflammation. The damage is associated with high myeloperoxidase activity, mainly as a reflection of neutrophilic infiltration into the damaged tissue (Veljaca et al., 1995) and caustic injury to the colonic epithelium and interstitium as measured by the rapid and dramatic increases in mucosal permeability (Yamada et al., 1992). It has been assumed that interstitial TNBS initiates the inflammatory response via macrophage-mediated recognition and degradation of TNBS-modified mucosal cells and proteins (Grisham et al., 1991). TNBS may reduce mucosal hydrophobicity by reacting with the surface-active phospholipids of the colonic mucosa. Reduced hydrophobic integrity of the colonic mucosa may contribute to TNBS-induced colonic inflammation (Tatsumi and Lichtenberger, 1996). TNBS causes necrosis and deeper tissue damage (somewhat akin to transmural inflammation seen in CD).

2.2 Adoptive transfer models

The adoptive transfer model involves transferring T cells or immune tissue from one mouse into a histocompatible, adoptive host which results in colitis. A variety of donors and hosts have been used, including CD4+ T cells transferred into severely immunodeficient (SCID) mice (Rudolphi et al., 1996), hsp60-specific CD8 + T-lymphocytes into $TCR^{-/-}$ or SCID mice (Steinhoff et al., 1999) and CD4+CD25- T cells into SCID mice (Kjellev et al., 2006).
Adoptive transfer models represent well-characterized models of chronic colitis induced by disruption of T cell homeostasis. The colitis is characterised by transmural inflammation, epithelial cell hyperplasia, polymorphonuclear leukocyte (PMN) and mononuclear leukocyte infiltration, crypt abscesses, and epithelial cell erosions. The disease model is responsive to a variety of treatment protocols (Ostanin et al., 2009). The adoptive host can influence the severity and location of colitis, with the recombinase activating gene-1-deficient ($RAG^{-/-}$) deficient mouse showing both small bowel inflammation and colitis, and therefore being the model most relevant for CD (Ostanin et al., 2009).
Because these models rely on the transfer of T cells, they are particularly useful in understanding how different T cell populations might contribute to the pathogenesis of IBD.

2.3 Genetic models of IBD

Recent research using novel genetic technologies has resulted in the identification of a large number of genes, variants of which may be related to increased susceptibility to IBD. Tools such as GWAS have identified susceptibility genes such as those encoding the autophagy protein ATG16L1, the receptor for prostaglandin E2 (CD), and the intestinal barrier protein ECM1 (UC) (Paul et al., 2011). Existing mouse and rat models containing relevant genetic variants, or those incorporating these newly identified variants, have been used to further investigate the genetic contribution to IBD. Gene variant models include knockouts (interleukin-2 KO/IL-2 receptor (R)α KO mice, T cell receptor (TCR) mutant mice, TNF-3′ untranslated region (UTR) KO mice, interleukin-22 KO mice) and transgenic models (IL-7 transgenic mice, signal transducer and activating transcription (STAT)-4 transgenic mice, HLA B27 transgenic rats), and have been comprehensively reviewed elsewhere (Jurjus et al., 2004; Mizoguchi and Mizoguchi, 2010). Some of these models develop spontaneous colitis as a result of the genetic variant, others can require additional intervention to act as a trigger for the onset of inflammation (Mizoguchi and Mizoguchi, 2010). For the purposes of this chapter, we will consider three models with which we have some experience; the interleukin 10 gene-deficient, multi-drug resistant gene-deficient, and *Nod2*^{2939iC} mouse models.

2.3.1 The interleukin 10 gene-deficient (*Il10*$^{-/-}$) mouse model

The *Il10*$^{-/-}$ mouse model has been widely used as a model of IBD (Kuhn et al., 1993; Berg, D. J. et al., 1996; Barnett et al., 2010). This mouse model lacks a functional version of the important anti-inflammatory cytokine interleukin 10. When originally developed, these mice were observed to be anaemic and underweight, and showed a chronic enterocolitis involving the entire intestinal tract. The intestinal pathology (Fig.1 [D–E]) was characterized by variable mucosal inflammation, abnormal crypt and villus structures, inflammatory cell infiltration and epithelial destruction (Kuhn et al., 1993).

The precise mechanism that results in inflammation in *Il10*$^{-/-}$ mice is unclear although, as is the case in human IBD, there is evidence of an inappropriate inflammatory response to normal intestinal flora (Sydora et al., 2003). This was seen in studies where mice raised in germ-free conditions showed no colitis (Sellon et al., 1998), while those under specific-pathogen free conditions showed a local colitis, and not the general enterocolitis seen in animals raised under conventional conditions (Kuhn et al., 1993). More specific studies of bacterial interactions have shown that clinical isolates of *Enterococcus faecalis* induce IBD-like symptoms in germ-free *Il10*$^{-/-}$ mice (Balish and Warner, 2002; Kim et al., 2005). Enterococcus species are a common component of the intestinal flora of healthy humans and animals (Jett et al., 1994), with *E. faecalis* and *E. faecium* being the most commonly detected species in the human bowel (Noble, 1978; Tannock and Cook, 2002). Both carry a variety of virulence factors which may play a role in the establishment of inflammation (Jett et al., 1994).

We have utilized *Il10*$^{-/-}$ mice inoculated with normal intestinal bacteria, including *Enterococcus* species (Barnett et al., 2010), to investigate the role of diet in intestinal inflammation. We have shown that food components such as polyunsaturated fatty acids (Knoch et al., 2009; Knoch et al., 2010) can prevent or ameliorate the level of intestinal inflammation, and have characterized changes in gene expression in association with this change in inflammation to better understand the mechanisms through which such food components might be acting.

We have also used metabolomic analysis to measure urinary metabolite differences between *Il10*$^{-/-}$ and wildtype C57BL/6 mice, and to determine which of these differences were associated with intestinal inflammation (Lin et al., 2010). Eleven metabolites, including glutaric acid, 2-hydroxyglutaric acid and 2-hydroxyadipic acid, were significantly different in *Il10*$^{-/-}$ compared with C57 mice, but these differences were not related to the severity of inflammation, and were possibly associated with the genetic manipulation that produced these animals, rather than any inflammatory-related function of IL-10. In contrast, fucose, xanthurenic acid and 5-aminovaleric acid were among fifteen metabolite differences associated with intestinal inflammation (Lin et al., 2010). The presence of defined metabolites associated with inflammation may be of benefit in enabling a non-invasive measurement of the severity of inflammation in human IBD.

2.3.2 The multi-drug resistant (Mdr1a) mouse model

Mdr1a (otherwise known as ATP-binding cassette, sub-family B (MDR/TAP), member 1A (Abcb1a)), is a member of a family of proteins that actively transport a wide range of

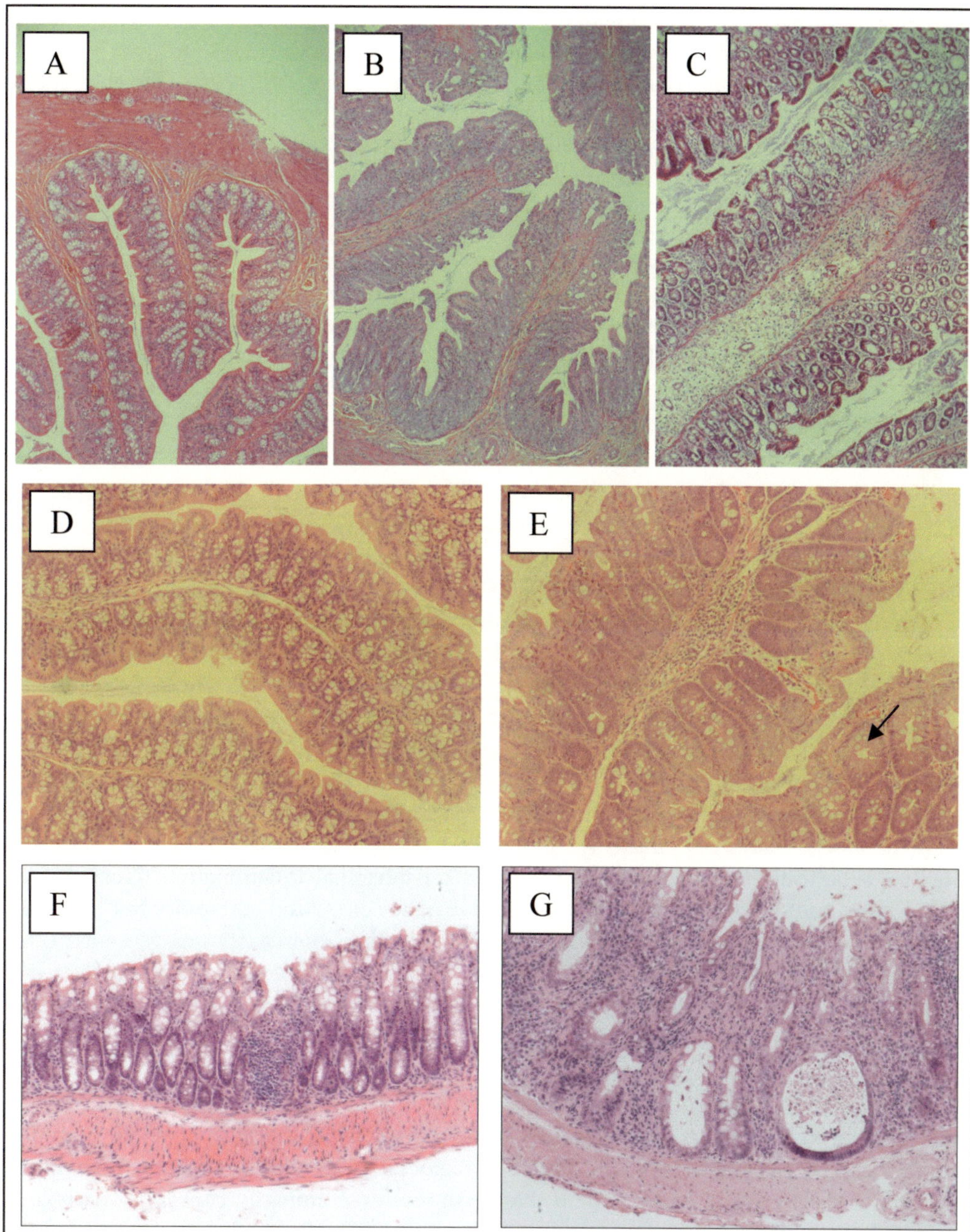

Fig. 1. Comparison of microscopic features of colon inflammation in a variety of animal models. DSS rat: Panels [A] to [C]. An untreated rat in panel [A] exhibits normal crypt distribution, high numbers of goblet cells, and intact surface enterocytes. There are noinflammatory aggregates, and immune cells present are well within normal limits. Sub mucosa and muscularis region are of normal size and proportion to the mucosa region. In a moderately inflamed colon [B], crypt loss, crypt shortening and aberrant crypts can be seen along with the associated loss of goblet cells, and some loss of integrity of the surface

enterocyte layer. An increasing number of inflammatory cells in the mucosa and submucosa region can also be seen. In a severely inflamed colon [C], the surface enterocyte layer is severely impaired. There is loss of crypts, and the majority of those still present are aberrant in structure, showing severe shortening. The number of goblet cells visible is significantly reduced and infiltrating inflammatory cells are evident throughout all definable regions of the tissue. Thickening/swelling/oedema of the submucosa region can also be observed.
Panel [D] shows a control C57 mouse which exhibits the intact enterocyte layer, abundant goblet cells, and normal crypt definition of a healthy mouse colon. In contract, the *Il10-/-* mouse in panel [E] shows aberrant crypts (black arrow) and crypt hyperplasia (swelling), an increase in inflammatory cells in the lamina propria and the presence of RBCs in the mucosa region of the tissue. There is also a decrease in goblet cell number and loss of surface enterocyte integrity. In panel [F], the FVB/N mouse is generally normal, although there is a lymphoid aggregate (arrow). In contrast, the Mdr1a mouse colon [G] shows significant inflammatory cell infiltration, aberrant crypts and some loss of surface enterocyte integrity

structurally unrelated, amphiphilic hydrophobic drugs from the cell, many of which are toxic compounds (Panwala et al., 1998). There is evidence that single nucleotide polymorphisms (SNPs) of the *MDR1* gene in the human population are associated with changes in the risk of UC (Huebner et al., 2009). Mice with a homozygous disruption of the *mdrla* gene were originally developed to better understand the physiological significance and other possible biological roles of this protein (Panwala et al., 1998). It was subsequently shown that these mice spontaneously develop intestinal inflammation (Fig.1, [F–G]) similar to that seen in human IBD, with infiltration of intestinal cells into the lamina propria, increased crypt length, goblet cell loss, interstitial oedema, ulceration (ranging from superficial to transmural) and crypt abscesses (Banner et al., 2004). These mice have since been used as an experimental model of colitis in a number of studies.
As in the case of the *Il10-/-* mice, we have used the Mdr1a mouse model to investigate potential beneficial effects of food components on intestinal inflammation (Nones et al., 2009). These studies have shown that the polyphenolic compound curcumin, but not rutin, significantly reduced colonic inflammation in Mdr1a mice. Microarray analyses suggested that curcumin reduced colon inflammation by up-regulating xenobiotic metabolism and down-regulating pro-inflammatory pathways, possibly through the pregnane X or retinoid X receptors (Nones et al., 2009).

2.3.3 The *Nod2^{2939iC}* mouse model

The NOD2 protein is important in the discrimination between normal intestinal flora and pathogenic bacteria (Inohara et al., 2002). It belongs to a class of pattern recognition receptors of the innate immune system that recognise evolutionarily conserved pathogen-associated molecular patterns. Pattern recognition by NOD2 initiates the signal transduction that leads to translocation of nuclear factor-kappa B (NF-κB) to the nucleus, transcription of specific genes and eventual activation of appropriate innate and adaptive immune responses (Inohara et al., 2002).
In humans, the most common CD susceptibility allele is 3020insC, which encodes a truncated NOD2 protein lacking the last 33 amino acids (Ogura et al., 2001). It has been established that this SNP, and possibly others in the *NOD2* gene, are important genetic determinants of CD risk in the NZ population (Leung et al., 2005). Variants of the NOD2

gene have also been shown to interact with other genes influencing bacterial recognition which results in an increased risk of IBD (Petermann et al., 2009a).
A mouse model has been generated containing a susceptibility allele homologous to that in humans (Maeda et al., 2005). These mice (*Nod2*^{2939iC}) express a protein truncated by 33 amino acids, which by itself does not alter the phenotype: homozygous *Nod2*^{2939iC} mice were healthy, not showing abnormalities of the gastrointestinal tract or other organs (Maeda et al., 2005). However, when 8-12 week old mice were exposed to DSS treatment (3% in drinking water), they exhibited increased body weight loss, increased colonic inflammation and ulceration and more apoptotic cells in the lamina propria when compared to similarly treated wild-type mice. The intestinal inflammatory response to DSS was dramatically reduced by oral antibiotics, suggesting that enteric bacteria elicit the inflammatory response to DSS, and without bacterial exposure, *Nod2*^{2939iC} mice have the same reaction as WT counterparts (Maeda et al., 2005).
We have inoculated these mice with intestinal bacteria, including *Enterococcus* strains, using the same protocol as previously applied to *Il10*$^{-/-}$ mice (Barnett et al., 2010). While there was some evidence of reduced body weight associated with the *Nod2*^{2939iC} mutation (WT > *Nod2*^{2939iC} heterozygotes > *Nod2*^{2939iC} homozygotes), there was no data to suggest an effect of either genotype or bacterial inoculation on intestinal phenotype, as assessed by assigning a histological injury score (Barnett et al, "unpublished observations"). It therefore seems likely that disruption of the epithelial barrier, for example with DSS, is necessary to enable bacterial infiltration which leads to altered NF-kB activation and IL-1β secretion in the *Nod2*^{2939iC} mice (Maeda et al., 2005).
This preliminary evidence suggests that the *Nod*^{22939iC} mutation is not, of itself, sufficient to lead to increased intestinal inflammation, requiring a simultaneous disruption of the epithelium. This is an example of an interaction between an environmental trigger, genetic susceptibility and inappropriate response to normal bacteria leading to intestinal inflammation. This model may therefore be particularly relevant for individuals in the human population carrying the homologous gene variant, and metabolomics approaches applied to this model may enable, for example, early detection of susceptibility to IBD and therefore earlier and more effective responses.

3. Lessons learned from mouse models

The body of evidence using mouse models of IBD is large, and there is no doubt that much has been learned by using such models. A selection of some key observations is shown in Table 1. This is clearly not an exhaustive list, but it serves to demonstrate some of the important areas in which animal models have contributed. In addition to more precisely defining the pathogenesis of IBD, insights have been gained into the inflammatory process itself, and this is relevant both in terms of colitis *per se* as well as being useful for the complications or systemic effects that may arise from a prolonged period of inflammation occurring within the intestine. There has also been progress in understanding the complex interactions occurring within the intestinal tract between the resident microbial population and the host.
Models such as the *Il10*$^{-/-}$ and adoptive transfer models have been particularly helpful in terms of generating deeper understanding of the inflammatory process itself. This has included better defining some of the leukoctye-epithelial cell interactions and the importance of cell adhesion, as well as the roles of the Th1 response in CD and the Th2 response (albeit an atypical one) in UC (Strober et al., 2002).

Model	Observation	Reference
TNBS	Fatty acid amide hydrolase (FAAH) inhibitors are promising targets for IBD treatment.	(Andrzejak et al., 2011)
DSS	DSS makes the inner colon mucus layer permeable to bacteria, which reach the epithelial cells and trigger an inflammatory reaction. Altered inner colon mucus layer may be an early event in colitis development.	(Johansson et al., 2010)
Various	IBD is much more complicated than currently predicted. Cell-specific, tissue-specific, or personalized approaches may be required for effective IBD therapy.	(Mizoguchi and Mizoguchi, 2010)
Various	A significant (as-yet not precisely defined) role for IL-10 in orchestrating intestinal immune homeostasis.	(Paul et al., 2011)
SAMP1/Yit	A hypothesis that CD is caused by a dysregulated immune response to an unknown (bacterial?) antigen in a genetically susceptible host.	(Pizarro et al., 2011)
TNFΔARE	Deregulation of TNF gene leads to spontaneous development of chronic ileitis similar to that of CD.	(Pizarro et al., 2011)
Various	Response in IBD takes the form of either a Th1 or Th2 T cell-mediated inflammation driven by antigens associated with normal mucosal microflora ("self" antigens).	(Strober et al., 2002)
Il10-/-	Importance of *Enterococcus* bacterial strains in development of intestinal inflammation.	(Balish and Warner, 2002; Barnett et al., 2010)
Il10-/-	Omega-3 and -6 polyunsatured fatty acids reduce intestinal inflammation in the *Il10-/-* mouse, in the case of n-3 via peroxisome proliferator-activated receptor a.	(Knoch et al., 2009; Knoch et al., 2010)
CD4+ SCID mice	Flagellins act as antigens that stimulate pathogenic intestinal immune reactions.	(Lodes et al., 2004)
Mdr1a	Reduction of inflammation associated with diets enriched with polyphenolic compounds.	(Nones et al., 2009)

Table 1. Some key observations from studies using mouse models of IBD

A variety of models have contributed to progress in understanding the complex interactions occurring within the intestinal tract between the resident microbial population and the host. A number of studies using *Il10-/-* mice have highlighted the importance of specific intestinal bacteria such as *Enterococcus* strains in triggering inflammation (Balish and Warner, 2002; Barnett et al., 2010). In terms of relevant components of bacteria which may be important, flagellins are molecules of the bacterial flagellum which are known to activate innate

immunity via toll-like receptor 5 (TLR5), and act as critical targets of the host's acquired immune system. These have been shown to elevated Th1 T cell responses in mice with colitis, and to thus be dominant antigens which may trigger the immune response in genetically susceptible individuals, leading to IBD (Lodes et al., 2004).
Potential therapeutic benefits include such molecules as superoxide dismutase 1 (SOD1), which has been shown to ameliorate colonic inflammatory changes in experimental colitis. Down-regulation of adhesion molecule expression, reduction of lipid hydroperoxidation, and recruitment of leukocytes into the inflamed intestine contribute to this beneficial effect (Segui et al., 2005). Our own studies have demonstrated the potential beneficial effects of dietary compounds such as polyunsaturated fatty acids (Knoch et al., 2009; Knoch et al., 2010) and polyphenols (Nones et al., 2009) on intestinal inflammation. A greater understanding of cell to cell adhesion has led to the development of monoclonal antibodies against α4 and α4β7 integrins that have been shown to have clinical efficacy (Lanzarotto et al., 2006), although there has been some debate as to the safety and efficacy of this approach (Davenport and Munday, 2007).

4. Relevance to the clinic

We will conclude our chapter by considering how information derived from these models has been applied to human IBD, and understanding both the value and limits of the lessons that have been learned from animal models. Finally, we will discuss the potential role of these models in the future of IBD research, and whether there are other alternatives to assist in translating fundamental research into a clinical setting.

4.1 Limits of animal models of IBD

Animal models can be an important tool in understanding complex diseases such as UC and CD, but it is important to remember that they are simply models. As such, they by definition will have some limitations, and while there are many similarities between experimental ulcerative disease of of the colon and human IBD, there are also differences. These can be either morphological (e.g., initial site of involvement of the bowel) or clinical. An example of a clinical difference is that spontaneous remission is sometimes seen in human disease (particularly with UC) but this is not seen in chemically-induced models unless exposure to the chemical is ceased. Mice may not be truly representative of other mammalian systems as has been observed with respect to early development (Berg, D. K. et al., 2011), and the inherent differences between mice and humans must be borne in mind when using such models.
The relevance of chemically-induced models has been called into question. It was noted early in the development of these models that there was a lack of any evidence that human ulcerative colitis is produced by the ingestion of compounds related to carrageenan, the chemical used to induce colitis (Watt and Marcus, 1973). Such evidence is still lacking, and it has also been observed that the acetic acid and TNBS models may have significant limitations in understanding events that initiate inflammation of the intestine in human IBD (Yamada et al., 1992). More recently, the relevance of the DSS-induced model has also been questioned (Petersen et al., 2009). To balance this, it should be noted that ulcerative disease of the colon can be caused by ingestion of certain chemical compounds in at least four different animal species, which suggests that this mechanism should not be completely disregarded with respect to human disease.

4.2 Application in a clinical setting

While animal models have clearly contributed to our knowledge of IBD, particularly in terms of understanding disease pathogenesis, the presence of useful progress in terms of treatment is less clear. There is an apparent lack of integration of mouse model data into the clinical setting, a so-called "missing link" between models and clinic (Petersen et al., 2009). This is seen in the conclusions to many studies incorporating such models, or indeed articles reviewing the use of these models, which tend to finish with statements referring to future, rather than current, therapeutic advances. Some examples of such conclusions are as follows (note that italics are not in the original references): "*...promising target* for the Inflammatory Bowel Diseases (IBD) treatment" (Andrzejak et al., 2011); "substantial investment from the pharmaceutical industry *should deliver* novel therapies arising from gene discovery to the clinic within the next 5 years" (Lees et al., 2011); "...recently established genetically engineered mouse models lacking IBD susceptibility gene *should be promising tools* to develop novel therapeutic measures for IBD" (Mizoguchi and Mizoguchi, 2010).

This is not to detract from some excellent research in the field, and the recently established genetically engineered mouse models lacking IBD susceptibility genes should indeed prove to be promising tools to develop novel therapies. For example, based on the numerous studies involving the *Il10*$^{-/-}$ mouse model demonstrating the importance of this anti-inflammatory cytokine in IBD, several human clinical trials have been carried out using IL-10. However, these have not shown a clear beneficial effect of IL-10 therapy. This has been attributed to polymorphisms of IL-10 receptors hampering effectiveness of this therapy for patients, or to the instability and short half-life of IL-10. More promisingly, engineered lactic acid bacteria have successfully delivered biologically active IL-10 into the intestine of both animal models (Wells and Mercenier, 2008) and some CD patients (Braat et al., 2006) indicating a potential bio-therapeutic application for IL-10.

4.3 Future relevance of animal models of IBD

It has been observed that differences between animal models may reflect the different subgroups of patients with IBD (Jurjus et al., 2004). This may be the case for some models, although the chemically-induced models may in fact be less relevant in terms of the clinical situation. Nevertheless, it seems clear that some of the genetically-based models may be of particular relevance for certain forms of IBD. In future, studies may utilise a specific mouse model targeted at the most appropriate subgroups and thus provide more relevant data. However, this will in turn rely on establishment of more clearly defined clinical phenotypes and the widespread application of genetic tests in clinical medicine to enable accurate matching of mouse model to patient thereby leading to the most appropriate therapy. The identification of appropriate diagnostic biomarkers would be of particular benefit in this case, both in terms of classification and subsequent monitoring of the effectiveness of therapies.

This potential 'matching' of model to patient sub-group may be constrained by financial considerations, nonetheless this personalised approach to treatment may be the most effective due to the heterogeneity of IBD. Recent evidence showing potential gene-diet interactions in IBD (Petermann et al., 2009b) and the potential for diet to modulate IBD through anti-inflammatory action or alteration of the microbiota (Issa and Saeian, 2011) suggests that dietary intervention appropriately matched to patient genotype may be an important aspect of successful therapy.

Mouse models will continue to be a pivotal part of IBD research. The complexity of the disease cannot currently be adequately modelled by *in vitro* or *in silico* approaches and requires an *in vivo* approach. Some novel therapies have shown promising initial data in limited human clinical trials, for example administration of viable eggs from the porcine whipworm, *Trichuris suis*, to patients with CD and UC, which may act to down-regulate the chronic Th1 immune response (Summers et al., 2003). However, more convincing safety and efficacy data derived from animal models are required before further human clinical trials using these novel treatments are conducted, particularly as some proposed treatments may have adverse effects on normal immune homeostasis (Grimm, 2009).

It has been observed that IBD may result from inappropriate responses to normal bacteria in a genetically susceptible host, which may arise due to some sort of environmental trigger. This situation is clearly seen in the *Nod2*^{2939iC} mouse, where the animals do not develop an inflammatory phenotype unless challenged with DSS, an insult which appears to damage the epithelial barrier and allow bacteria to infiltrate the mucosa, leading to an inappropriate response in the *Nod2*^{2939iC}, but not the wild-type, mouse. The requirement for a trigger in the form of DSS may make this model more relevant, as it could reflect the situation seen in human patients with this gene variant, who may have been exposed to some form of intestinal insult (dietary, or an infection) which has enabled the interaction with bacteria to occur. However, the fact that DSS is the trigger could be a weakness; as already observed, this particular compound has been questioned in terms of its relevance, and it may be that a more relevant trigger (e.g. dietary) needs to be found before such a model could be truly relevant.

The current comprehensive knowledge of the potential genetic component of both CD and UC, and rapid decreases in the cost of techniques to accurately measure these on an individual level, mean that more accurate classification of disease based on both clinical and genetic factors is achievable. The presence of multiple animal models, which may reflect these more accurately classified subgroups, means that a more targeted use of these models can be made. There is a growing body of evidence on the interactions between drugs (pharmacogenomics) or foods (nutrigenomics) and an individual's genotype. A truly personalised approach to managing IBD using appropriate preventive or therapeutic pharmacological or nutritional interventions is a future prospect if continued advances are made in this area.

In summary, there is clearly still a role for animal models of IBD, however more appropriate use of new information and technologies, better classification of IBD based on both phenotypic and genetic information, and closer alliances between fundamental biological researchers and clinicians are required to ensure that the key lessons from these models are effectively moved into clinical practice. This should enable more successful strategies for the prevention and amelioration of this debilitating condition.

5. Acknowledgment

The authors wish to thank Virginia Parslow and Drs Emma Bermingham and Nicole Roy for constructive criticism of this work, Shuotun Zhu for supplying Mdr1a mouse histology images, and Kelly Armstrong for supplying DSS rat and *Il10*$^{-/-}$ mouse histology images, and the associated descriptions of inflammation. This work is associated with the Nutrigenomics New Zealand (NuNZ) collaboration between The University of Auckland, AgResearch

Limited, and Plant & Food Research, and is partly funded by the New Zealand Ministry of Science and Innovation.

6. References

Abraham, C. & Cho, J. H. (2009). Inflammatory Bowel Disease, *New England Journal of Medicine*, Vol.361, No.21, pp. 2066-2078.

Alex, P.; Zachos, N. C.; Nguyen, T.; Gonzales, L.; Chen, T. E.; Conklin, L. S.; Centola, M. & Li, X. (2009). Distinct cytokine patterns identified from multiplex profiles of murine DSS and TNBS-induced colitis, *Inflamm Bowel Dis*, Vol.15, No.3, pp. 341-52.

Andrzejak, V.; Muccioli, G. G.; Body-Malapel, M. et al. (2011). New FAAH inhibitors based on 3-carboxamido-5-aryl-isoxazole scaffold that protect against experimental colitis, *Bioorg Med Chem*, Vol.19, No.12, pp. 3777-86.

Balish, E. & Warner, T. (2002). Enterococcus faecalis induces inflammatory bowel disease in interleukin-10 knockout mice, *Am J Pathol*, Vol.160, No.6, pp. 2253-7.

Banner, K. H.; Cattaneo, C.; Le Net, J. L.; Popovic, A.; Collins, D. & Gale, J. D. (2004). Macroscopic, microscopic and biochemical characterisation of spontaneous colitis in a transgenic mouse, deficient in the multiple drug resistance 1a gene, *Br J Pharmacol*, Vol.143, No.5, pp. 590-8.

Barnett, M. P.; McNabb, W. C.; Cookson, A. L. et al. (2010). Changes in colon gene expression associated with increased colon inflammation in interleukin-10 gene-deficient mice inoculated with Enterococcus species, *BMC Immunol*, Vol.11, pp. 39.

Barrett, J. C.; Hansoul, S.; Nicolae, D. L. et al. (2008). Genome-wide association defines more than 30 distinct susceptibility loci for Crohn's disease, *Nat Genet*, Vol.40, No.8, pp. 955-62.

Berg, D. J.; Davidson, N.; Kuhn, R. et al. (1996). Enterocolitis and colon cancer in interleukin-10-deficient mice are associated with aberrant cytokine production and CD4(+) TH1-like responses, *J Clin Invest*, Vol.98, No.4, pp. 1010-20.

Berg, D. K.; Smith, C. S.; Pearton, D. J.; Wells, D. N.; Broadhurst, R.; Donnison, M. & Pfeffer, P. L. (2011). Trophectoderm lineage determination in cattle, *Dev Cell*, Vol.20, No.2, pp. 244-55.

Braat, H.; Rottiers, P.; Hommes, D. W. et al. (2006). A phase I trial with transgenic bacteria expressing interleukin-10 in Crohn's disease, *Clin Gastroenterol Hepatol*, Vol.4, No.6, pp. 754-9.

Brest, P.; Corcelle, E. A.; Cesaro, A. et al. (2010). Autophagy and Crohn's disease: at the crossroads of infection, inflammation, immunity, and cancer, *Curr Mol Med*, Vol.10, No.5, pp. 486-502.

Burstein, M.; Scholnick, H. R. & Morfin, R. (1970). Rapid method for the isolation of lipoproteins from human serum by precipitation with polyanions, *J Lipid Res*, Vol.11, No.6, pp. 583-95.

Cosnes, J.; Gower-Rousseau, C.; Seksik, P. & Cortot, A. (2011). Epidemiology and natural history of inflammatory bowel diseases, *Gastroenterology*, Vol.140, No.6, pp. 1785-94.

Davenport, R. J. & Munday, J. R. (2007). Alpha4-integrin antagonism--an effective approach for the treatment of inflammatory diseases?, *Drug Discov Today*, Vol.12, No.13-14, pp. 569-76.

Depoortere, I.; Thijs, T.; Keith, J., Jr. & Peeters, T. L. (2004). Treatment with interleukin-11 affects plasma leptin levels in inflamed and non-inflamed rabbits, *Regul Pept*, Vol.122, No.3, pp. 149-56.

Grimm, M. C. (2009). New and emerging therapies for inflammatory bowel diseases, *J Gastroenterol Hepatol*, Vol.24 Suppl 3, pp. S69-74.

Grisham, M. B.; Volkmer, C.; Tso, P. & Yamada, T. (1991). Metabolism of trinitrobenzene sulfonic acid by the rat colon produces reactive oxygen species, *Gastroenterology*, Vol.101, No.2, pp. 540-7.

Halfvarson, J.; Bodin, L.; Tysk, C.; Lindberg, E. & Jarnerot, G. (2003). Inflammatory bowel disease in a Swedish twin cohort: a long-term follow-up of concordance and clinical characteristics, *Gastroenterology*, Vol.124, No.7, pp. 1767-73.

Huebner, C.; Browning, B. L.; Petermann, I. et al. (2009). Genetic analysis of MDR1 and inflammatory bowel disease reveals protective effect of heterozygous variants for ulcerative colitis, *Inflamm Bowel Dis*, Vol.15, No.12, pp. 1784-93.

Inohara, N.; Ogura, Y. & Nunez, G. (2002). Nods: a family of cytosolic proteins that regulate the host response to pathogens, *Curr Opin Microbiol*, Vol.5, No.1, pp. 76-80.

Ishioka, T.; Kuwabara, N.; Oohashi, Y. & Wakabayashi, K. (1987). Induction of colorectal tumors in rats by sulfated polysaccharides, *Crit Rev Toxicol*, Vol.17, No.3, pp. 215-44.

Issa, M. & Saeian, K. (2011). Diet in inflammatory bowel disease, *Nutr Clin Pract*, Vol.26, No.2, pp. 151-4.

Jett, B. D.; Huycke, M. M. & Gilmore, M. S. (1994). Virulence of enterococci, *Clin Microbiol Rev*, Vol.7, No.4, pp. 462-78.

Johansson, M. E.; Gustafsson, J. K.; Sjoberg, K. E.; Petersson, J.; Holm, L.; Sjovall, H. & Hansson, G. C. (2010). Bacteria penetrate the inner mucus layer before inflammation in the dextran sulfate colitis model, *PLoS One*, Vol.5, No.8, pp. e12238.

Jurjus, A. R.; Khoury, N. N. & Reimund, J. M. (2004). Animal models of inflammatory bowel disease, *J Pharmacol Toxicol Methods*, Vol.50, No.2, pp. 81-92.

Juyal, G.; Prasad, P.; Senapati, S.; Midha, V.; Sood, A.; Amre, D.; Juyal, R. C. & Thelma, B. K. (2011). An investigation of genome-wide studies reported susceptibility loci for ulcerative colitis shows limited replication in north Indians, *PLoS One*, Vol.6, No.1, pp. e16565.

Kent, P. W.; Hichens, M. & Ward, P. F. V. (1958). Displacement fractionation of deoxyribonucleoproteins by heparin and dextran sulphate., *Biochemical Journal*, Vol.68, pp. 568-572.

Kim, S. C.; Tonkonogy, S. L.; Albright, C. A.; Tsang, J.; Balish, E. J.; Braun, J.; Huycke, M. M. & Sartor, R. B. (2005). Variable phenotypes of enterocolitis in interleukin 10-deficient mice monoassociated with two different commensal bacteria, *Gastroenterology*, Vol.128, No.4, pp. 891-906.

Kjellev, S.; Lundsgaard, D.; Poulsen, S. S. & Markholst, H. (2006). Reconstitution of Scid mice with CD4+CD25- T cells leads to rapid colitis: an improved model for pharmacologic testing, *Int Immunopharmacol*, Vol.6, No.8, pp. 1341-54.

Knoch, B.; Barnett, M. P.; McNabb, W. C.; Zhu, S.; Park, Z. A.; Khan, A. & Roy, N. C. (2010). Dietary arachidonic acid-mediated effects on colon inflammation using transcriptome analysis, *Mol Nutr Food Res*, Vol.54 Suppl 1, pp. S62-74.

Knoch, B.; Barnett, M. P.; Zhu, S. et al. (2009). Genome-wide analysis of dietary eicosapentaenoic acid- and oleic acid-induced modulation of colon inflammation in interleukin-10 gene-deficient mice, *J Nutrigenet Nutrigenomics*, Vol.2, No.1, pp. 9-28.

Kocak, E.; Koklu, S.; Akbal, E.; Tas, A.; Karaca, G.; Astarci, M. H.; Guven, B. & Can, M. (2011). NaOH-Induced Crohn's Colitis in Rats: A Novel Experimental Model, *Dig Dis Sci*, pp.

Kuhn, R.; Lohler, J.; Rennick, D.; Rajewsky, K. & Muller, W. (1993). Interleukin-10-deficient mice develop chronic enterocolitis, *Cell*, Vol.75, No.2, pp. 263-74.

Lanzarotto, F.; Carpani, M.; Chaudhary, R. & Ghosh, S. (2006). Novel treatment options for inflammatory bowel disease: targeting alpha 4 integrin, *Drugs*, Vol.66, No.9, pp. 1179-89.

Lees, C. W.; Barrett, J. C.; Parkes, M. & Satsangi, J. (2011). New IBD genetics: common pathways with other diseases, *Gut*, pp.

Leung, E.; Hong, J.; Fraser, A. G.; Merriman, T. R.; Vishnu, P.; Abbott, W. G. & Krissansen, G. W. (2005). Polymorphisms of CARD15/NOD2 and CD14 genes in New Zealand Crohn's disease patients, *Immunol Cell Biol*, Vol.83, No.5, pp. 498-503.

Lin, H. M.; Barnett, M. P.; Roy, N. C. et al. (2010). Metabolomic analysis identifies inflammatory and noninflammatory metabolic effects of genetic modification in a mouse model of Crohn's disease, *J Proteome Res*, Vol.9, No.4, pp. 1965-75.

Lodes, M. J.; Cong, Y.; Elson, C. O.; Mohamath, R.; Landers, C. J.; Targan, S. R.; Fort, M. & Hershberg, R. M. (2004). Bacterial flagellin is a dominant antigen in Crohn disease, *J Clin Invest*, Vol.113, No.9, pp. 1296-306.

MacPherson, B. R. & Pfeiffer, C. J. (1978). Experimental production of diffuse colitis in rats, *Digestion*, Vol.17, No.2, pp. 135-50.

Maeda, S.; Hsu, L. C.; Liu, H.; Bankston, L. A.; Iimura, M.; Kagnoff, M. F.; Eckmann, L. & Karin, M. (2005). Nod2 mutation in Crohn's disease potentiates NF-kappaB activity and IL-1beta processing, *Science*, Vol.307, No.5710, pp. 734-8.

Mahurkar, S.; Banerjee, R.; Rani, V. S.; Thakur, N.; Rao, G. V.; Reddy, D. N. & Chandak, G. R. (2010). Common variants in NOD2 and IL23R are not associated with inflammatory bowel disease in Indians, *J Gastroenterol Hepatol*, Vol.26, No.4, pp. 694-9.

Marcus, R. & Watt, J. (1969). Seaweeds and ulcerative colitis in laboratory animals, *Lancet*, Vol.2, No.7618, pp. 489-90.

Massey, D. C. & Parkes, M. (2007). Genome-wide association scanning highlights two autophagy genes, ATG16L1 and IRGM, as being significantly associated with Crohn's disease, *Autophagy*, Vol.3, No.6, pp. 649-51.

Mizoguchi, A. & Mizoguchi, E. (2010). Animal models of IBD: linkage to human disease, *Curr Opin Pharmacol*, Vol.10, No.5, pp. 578-87.

Moyana, T. N. & Lalonde, J. M. (1990). Carrageenan-induced intestinal injury in the rat--a model for inflammatory bowel disease, *Ann Clin Lab Sci*, Vol.20, No.6, pp. 420-6.

Nakagome, S.; Takeyama, Y.; Mano, S.; Sakisaka, S.; Matsui, T.; Kawamura, S. & Oota, H. (2010). Population-specific susceptibility to Crohn's disease and ulcerative colitis; dominant and recessive relative risks in the Japanese population, *Ann Hum Genet*, Vol.74, No.2, pp. 126-36.

Nell, S.; Suerbaum, S. & Josenhans, C. (2010). The impact of the microbiota on the pathogenesis of IBD: lessons from mouse infection models, *Nat Rev Microbiol*, Vol.8, No.8, pp. 564-77.

Noble, C. J. (1978). Carriage of group D streptococci in the human bowel, *J Clin Pathol*, Vol.31, No.12, pp. 1182-6.

Nones, K.; Dommels, Y. E.; Martell, S. et al. (2009). The effects of dietary curcumin and rutin on colonic inflammation and gene expression in multidrug resistance gene-deficient (mdr1a-/-) mice, a model of inflammatory bowel diseases, *Br J Nutr*, Vol.101, No.2, pp. 169-81.

Ogura, Y.; Bonen, D. K.; Inohara, N. et al. (2001). A frameshift mutation in NOD2 associated with susceptibility to Crohn's disease, *Nature*, Vol.411, No.6837, pp. 603-6.

Okayasu, I.; Hatakeyama, S.; Yamada, M.; Ohkusa, T.; Inagaki, Y. & Nakaya, R. (1990). A novel method in the induction of reliable experimental acute and chronic ulcerative colitis in mice, *Gastroenterology*, Vol.98, No.3, pp. 694-702.

Ostanin, D. V.; Bao, J.; Koboziev, I.; Gray, L.; Robinson-Jackson, S. A.; Kosloski-Davidson, M.; Price, V. H. & Grisham, M. B. (2009). T cell transfer model of chronic colitis: concepts, considerations, and tricks of the trade, *Am J Physiol Gastrointest Liver Physiol*, Vol.296, No.2, pp. G135-46.

Panwala, C. M.; Jones, J. C. & Viney, J. L. (1998). A novel model of inflammatory bowel disease: mice deficient for the multiple drug resistance gene, mdr1a, spontaneously develop colitis, *J Immunol*, Vol.161, No.10, pp. 5733-44.

Paul, G.; Khare, V. & Gasche, C. (2011). Inflamed gut mucosa: downstream of interleukin-10, *Eur J Clin Invest*, pp.

Petermann, I.; Huebner, C.; Browning, B. L. et al. (2009a). Interactions among genes influencing bacterial recognition increase IBD risk in a population-based New Zealand cohort, *Hum Immunol*, Vol.70, No.6, pp. 440-6.

Petermann, I.; Triggs, C. M.; Huebner, C. et al. (2009b). Mushroom intolerance: a novel diet-gene interaction in Crohn's disease, *Br J Nutr*, Vol.102, No.4, pp. 506-8.

Petersen, Y. M.; Björkenberg, B.; Christjansen, K.; Stahlhut, M.; Pedersen, H. D. & Thorkildsen, C. (2009). Is the murine dextran sodium sulfate-induced colitis model valid for predicting drug efficacy in IBD?, *Digestive Diseases Week*, pp.

Pizarro, T. T.; Pastorelli, L.; Bamias, G. et al. (2011). SAMP1/YitFc mouse strain: A spontaneous model of Crohn's disease-like ileitis, *Inflamm Bowel Dis*, pp.

Rudolphi, A.; Bonhagen, K. & Reimann, J. (1996). Polyclonal expansion of adoptively transferred CD4+ alpha beta T cells in the colonic lamina propria of scid mice with colitis, *Eur J Immunol*, Vol.26, No.5, pp. 1156-63.

Sanchez-Munoz, F.; Dominguez-Lopez, A. & Yamamoto-Furusho, J. K. (2008). Role of cytokines in inflammatory bowel disease, *World J Gastroenterol*, Vol.14, No.27, pp. 4280-8.

Segui, J.; Gil, F.; Gironella, M. et al. (2005). Down-regulation of endothelial adhesion molecules and leukocyte adhesion by treatment with superoxide dismutase is beneficial in chronic immune experimental colitis, *Inflamm Bowel Dis*, Vol.11, No.10, pp. 872-82.

Sellon, R. K.; Tonkonogy, S.; Schultz, M.; Dieleman, L. A.; Grenther, W.; Balish, E.; Rennick, D. M. & Sartor, R. B. (1998). Resident enteric bacteria are necessary for development of spontaneous colitis and immune system activation in interleukin-10-deficient mice, *Infect Immun*, Vol.66, No.11, pp. 5224-31.

Shibata, Y.; Taruishi, M. & Ashida, T. (1993). Experimental ileitis in dogs and colitis in rats with trinitrobenzene sulfonic acid--colonoscopic and histopathologic studies, *Gastroenterol Jpn*, Vol.28, No.4, pp. 518-27.

Steinhoff, U.; Brinkmann, V.; Klemm, U. et al. (1999). Autoimmune intestinal pathology induced by hsp60-specific CD8 T cells, *Immunity*, Vol.11, No.3, pp. 349-58.

Strober, W.; Fuss, I. J. & Blumberg, R. S. (2002). The immunology of mucosal models of inflammation, *Annu Rev Immunol*, Vol.20, pp. 495-549.

Summers, R. W.; Elliott, D. E.; Qadir, K.; Urban, J. F., Jr.; Thompson, R. & Weinstock, J. V. (2003). Trichuris suis seems to be safe and possibly effective in the treatment of inflammatory bowel disease, *Am J Gastroenterol*, Vol.98, No.9, pp. 2034-41.

Sydora, B. C.; Tavernini, M. M.; Wessler, A.; Jewell, L. D. & Fedorak, R. N. (2003). Lack of interleukin-10 leads to intestinal inflammation, independent of the time at which luminal microbial colonization occurs, *Inflamm Bowel Dis*, Vol.9, No.2, pp. 87-97.

Tannock, G. W. & Cook, G. (2002). Enterococci as members of the intestinal microflora of humans, *The enterococci: pathogenesis, molecular biology, and antibiotic resistance*, pp. 101-132.

Tatsumi, Y. & Lichtenberger, L. M. (1996). Molecular association of trinitrobenzenesulfonic acid and surface phospholipids in the development of colitis in rats, *Gastroenterology*, Vol.110, No.3, pp. 780-9.

Thompson, A. I. & Lees, C. W. (2011). Genetics of ulcerative colitis, *Inflamm Bowel Dis*, Vol.17, No.3, pp. 831-48.

Tsianos, E. V. & Katsanos, K. (2009). Do we really understand what the immunological disturbances in inflammatory bowel disease mean?, *World J Gastroenterol*, Vol.15, No.5, pp. 521-5.

Van Limbergen, J.; Wilson, D. C. & Satsangi, J. (2009). The genetics of Crohn's disease, *Annu Rev Genomics Hum Genet*, Vol.10, pp. 89-116.

Veljaca, M.; Lesch, C. A.; Pllana, R.; Sanchez, B.; Chan, K. & Guglietta, A. (1995). BPC-15 reduces trinitrobenzene sulfonic acid-induced colonic damage in rats, *J Pharmacol Exp Ther*, Vol.272, No.1, pp. 417-22.

Wahl, G. M.; Stern, M. & Stark, G. R. (1979). Efficient transfer of large DNA fragments from agarose gels to diazobenzyloxymethyl-paper and rapid hybridization by using dextran sulfate, *Proc Natl Acad Sci U S A*, Vol.76, No.8, pp. 3683-7.

Watt, J. & Marcus, R. (1973). Experimental ulcerative disease of the colon in animals, *Gut*, Vol.14, No.6, pp. 506-10.

Wells, J. M. & Mercenier, A. (2008). Mucosal delivery of therapeutic and prophylactic molecules using lactic acid bacteria, *Nat Rev Microbiol*, Vol.6, No.5, pp. 349-62.

Yamada, Y.; Marshall, S.; Specian, R. D. & Grisham, M. B. (1992). A comparative analysis of two models of colitis in rats, *Gastroenterology*, Vol.102, No.5, pp. 1524-34.